VOLUME 4

COMPREHENSIVE NEUROLOGIC REHABILITATION

MULTIPLE SCLEROSIS

A REHABILITATION APPROACH TO MANAGEMENT

RANDALL T. SCHAPIRO, MD

Fairview Multiple Sclerosis Center
Riverside Medical Center
and
Clinical Professor of Neurology
University of Minnesota
Minneapolis, MN

Demos Publications, 156 Fifth Avenue, New York, NY 10010

Made in the United States of America.

ISBN: 0-939957-37-X
LC: 91-073106

PREFACE

Multiple sclerosis is the most common chronic, nontraumatic neurologic disease of young adults. While no therapy exists to "cure" the disease, much can be done to manage its symptoms and to permit most patients to lead relatively normal lives. The techniques of rehabilitation that can be successfully applied to the management of the disease may involve specialists from a variety of fields, including physical and occupational therapy, neurology, physiatry, and speech pathology.

This book was designed to aid in the understanding of the various rehabilitation techniques available to the health professional working with people who have MS. Despite the fact that rehabilitation techniques are often highly effective, little documentation and research exists to provide a scientific basis for their application to these patients. Treatment to date has therefore been highly empirical. The contributors to this volume all have extensive experience with the disease, and the practical techniques that they have found useful are presented in detail.

The text is organized into sections based on the professions of neurology, occupational therapy, physical therapy, and speech pathology. While rehabilitation utilizes a team approach, and divisions among specialties may be less formal than in other medical settings, the decision to organize the book in this manner was based on the very real divisions of expertise and practice that exist in many or most institutions. There is as a result a certain amount of repetition among sections, albeit with important differences of perspective. For example, occupational therapy traditionally deals with problems of the upper extremities, physical therapy with the lower; thus spasticity, balance, and coordination are discussed in both sections.

The scope of rehabilitation may be described in very broad or very narrow terms. We have taken essentially a middle course. Areas of rehabilitation that tend to utilize a more pharmacologic approach, such as bladder and bowel management, have not been included. Nor have we included an extensive discussion of the cognitive problems now known to be in some degree widespread in MS, since their practical rehabilitation remains sadly lacking. While no formal chapter exists on motivation, its importance is sprinkled throughout the book.

Psychological, social, and marital problems are also common in MS, and the reader will find numerous comments directed to rehabilitation professionals concerning their role in this complex area. By necessity, these are superficial. However, everyone involved in rehabilitation should appreciate the importance of these problems and their impact on the overall rehabilitation process.

MS is more than a unique disease. Each individual with the disease is unique, given the virtually infinite combinations of abnormalities that can occur dependent upon the pattern of lesion formation. This fact prohibits the development of a set rehabilitation program for everyone with the disease. Hopefully, this text will contain "pearls" of unique knowledge that will allow the reader to develop individualized rehabilitation programs for those with MS. However, the bulk of the book is practical rehabilitation viewed from the perspective of those who work on an ongoing basis with MS persons.

ACKNOWLEDGMENTS

A debt of gratitude is owed to many but all of us associated with this book want to thank our patients who, in the end, have taught us the substance of the material we hope to teach others. A special thanks goes to Diana M. Schneider, Ph.D. (Demos) for her help and encouragement with the manuscript.

CONTRIBUTORS

The many contributors to this volume deserve special acknowlegment for their research contributions, and for sharing their wealth of professional experiences upon which these pages are based.

JULIE ARNDT, B.S., R.P.T.
Fairview MS Center
Riverside Medical Center
Minneapolis, Minnesota

CHARLOTTE BHASIN, M.O.T., O.T.R./L
The Mellen Center for Research and Treatment in MS
Cleveland Clinic Foundation
Cleveland, Ohio

SURINDER P. BRAR, B.S., R.P.T
The Rocky Mountain MS Center
Swedish Hospital
Denver, Colorado

ROBERT HABASEVICH, M.S., R.P.T.
Moss Rehabilitation
Philadelphia, Pennsylvania
and The Jimmie Heuga Center
Vail, Colorado

JANIS JACOBS, M.S., L.P.T.
The Mellen Center for Research and Treatment in MS
Cleveland Clinic Foundation
Cleveland, Ohio

DONNA JENSEN, O.T.R.
Fairview MS Center
Riverside Medical Center
Minneapolis, Minnesota

CAROL KLITZKE, M.A., C.C.C./S.L.P.
Fairview MS Center
Riverside Medical Center
Minneapolis, Minnesota

MARY LENLING, O.T.R.
Fairview MS Center
Riverside Medical Center
Minneapolis, Minnesota

KATE ROBBINS, O.T.R.
The Albert Einstein MS Center
Bronx, New York

ANDREA SELZER-SILVERMAN, O.T.R.
Fairview MS Center
Riverside Medical Center
Minneapolis, Minnesota

KAREN TARBUCK-NELSON, B.S., R.P.T.
Fairview MS Center
Riverside Medical Center
Minneapolis, Minnesota

JULIE VARNO, M.S., R.P.T.
Fairview MS Center
Riverside Medical Center
Minneapolis, Minnesota

CONTENTS

1

THE NEUROLOGIC BASIS OF MULTIPLE SCLEROSIS

RANDALL T. SCHAPIRO, M.D.

Multiple sclerosis (MS) is a disease of the central nervous system (CNS) involving myelin and the cells that produce it, the oligodendroglia. Myelin is the relatively complex "insulation" of axons, composed primarily of lipid and protein. Demyelination occurs predominantly along the walls of the ventricles of the brain. Cells of the immune system invade and destroy the myelin, allowing other CNS cells, the astroglia, to produce a scar (plaque) around the multiple demyelinating sites. Thus the name *multiple sclerosis,* meaning "multiple hardened scars," is appropriate.

Although the cause of MS remains a mystery, a number of observations have lead to several different hypotheses.

1

EPIDEMIOLOGY OF MULTIPLE SCLEROSIS

• Multiple sclerosis appears more prominently in areas of the world away from the equator, both north and south of the equator. This may be due to climatic, environmental, or sanitary conditions, or simply to the fact that certain ethnic groups live in these areas. Northern Europeans and their descendents appear to have a higher incidence of MS.

• A second observation, which further complicates the first, is that the location where a person spends his/her first fifteen years of life (north or south) determines a greater or lesser likelihood of developing MS. A person born in the north who moves to the south after age 15 is more likely to develop MS than one who moves south to north. The prevalence rate for MS in the northern United States is over 100/100,000 population versus 30/100,000 in the southern United States.

• The Shetland and Orkney Islands (British), off the coast of Scotland, have a prevalence for MS of 450/100,000. Adjacent islands, the Faroe Islands (Danish), had little MS until World War II, when the rate began to match that of the Shetlands and Orkneys coincident with the British troops occupying the Faroes. Why MS increased is not clear, but the rate again decreased six years after the troops left.

PROSPECT OF A VIRUS

These facts among others suggest a viral etiology, but a number of different leads remain unproven. There is evidence of increased amounts of various viral particles, antibodies, and other signs of viral infection in the cerebrospinal fluid (CSF) of people with MS. Despite this evidence, no virus has clearly been associated with or consistently isolated from those with MS. Each decade has had a virus linked to MS: the measles virus in the 1970s and herpes in the 1980s. In the 1990s, a new candidate has appeared, a retrovirus peripherally related to that which produces AIDS, classified as the HTLV-I virus. This virus is an attractive candidate because it is involved in another demyelinating disease, tropical spastic paraparesis (TSP). The studies linking MS to the HTLV-I virus need further review but are intriguing. A viral inter-action is an attractive hypothesis.

IMMUNE SYSTEM AND HEREDITY

It appears fairly clear that a disorder of the immune system is involved in this disease. The cellular components of the immune sys-tem, T and B cells, are involved in a variety of different ways in MS. Why or how the immune system is altered remains a major question. Heredity is almost certainly a factor in MS etiology. Facts that implicate genetics include the following:

- MS appears more predominantly in women (1.8:1).
- MS is seen predominantly in whites.
- MS is more frequent in certain human leukocyte antigen (HLA) tis-sue types. HLA typing became popular with the transplant revolu-tion and is a means of examining the genetic components of chro-mosome 6. These become markers and become popular tools in the analysis of genetics. While not conclusive, these data strongly sug-gest that certain HLA-typed individuals are more likely to develop MS than others.

Thus, the cause of MS is probably multifactorial; an individual may be predisposed to develop MS if the appropriate combination of factors exist. For example s/he may inherit an immune system which may be triggered by a virus or similar organism to attack the myelin and/or oligodendroglial cell. Over time, the multiple scars resulting from this process yield the clinical picture of MS.

DIAGNOSIS OF MULTIPLE SCLEROSIS

While the cause of MS remains a mystery, the ability to diag-nose the process has improved markedly in the past few years. There remain four basic clinical tenants to the diagnosis:

1. The disease usually has its onset between the ages of 15 and 50.
2. Its course usually fluctuates, with exacerbations followed by remissions in which the patient stabilizes or improves.
3. There are usually multiple abnormalities within the CNS.
4. There is no other readily obvious explanation for the neurological picture, e.g., metastatic cancer, vasculitis, or multiple vascular infarcts.

A number of diagnostic tests aid in confirming the diagnosis (Fig. 1.1). Evoked potential measurements test the spread and efficiency of

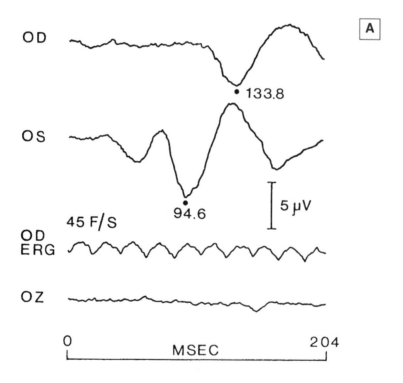

FIGURE. 1.1. A: Pattern shift visual evoked response demonstrating the delay in conduction often seen in MS. B: MRI of the head demonstrating the abnormalities seen in MS.

conduction within the CNS (Fig. 1.1A). The CSF can be evaluated for myelin breakdown products and evidence of immune system dysfunction, including myelin basic protein and oligoclonal banding of IgG. Magnetic resonance imaging (MRI) has revolutionized the imaging of the nervous system, especially the demyelinating nervous system (Fig. 1.1B). The changes of water content in the regions attacked immunologically allow changes in the MRI scan which are obvious and thus visualization of abnormalities within the myelin occurs. The diagnosis of MS has become much easier since these diagnostic tools have been added to the clinical examination.

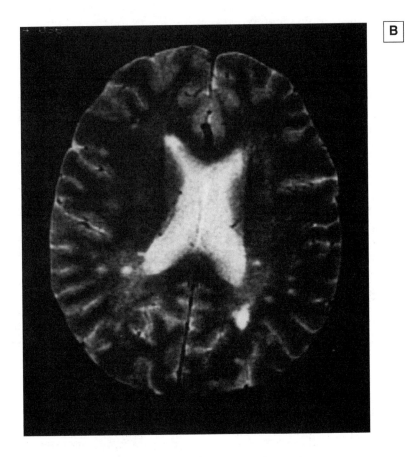

TYPES OF MULTIPLE SCLEROSIS

Depending on the progression of clinical symptoms, MS may be classified into five fairly distinct types (Fig. 1.2):

1. Benign MS, which develops little progression (Fig. 1.2A).
2. Benign relapsing-remitting disease, which presents with fluctuations of symptoms and only mild disability (Fig. 1.2B).
3. Chronic relapsing MS, which is indicated by significantly increasing disability with each attack (Fig. 1.2C).
4. Chronic progressive MS, which is characterized by a lack of remission with continued progressive disability.

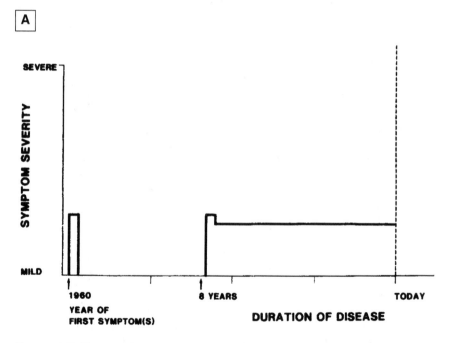

FIGURE 1.2. Progression of disease over time. **A:** Benign MS leads to very little disability. **B:** Benign relapsing-remitting MS leads to little disability. **C:** Chronic relapsing progressive MS leads to significant disability. **D:** Chronic progressive MS leads to very significant disability. **E:** Acute progressive MS quickly leads to very significant disability.

5. Acute progressive MS, which is defined by a rapid progression to disability.

In the aggregate, two thirds of the people with known MS remain ambulatory and functional after 20 years. Thus, a diagnosis of MS is clearly not a mandatory sentence to a wheelchair.

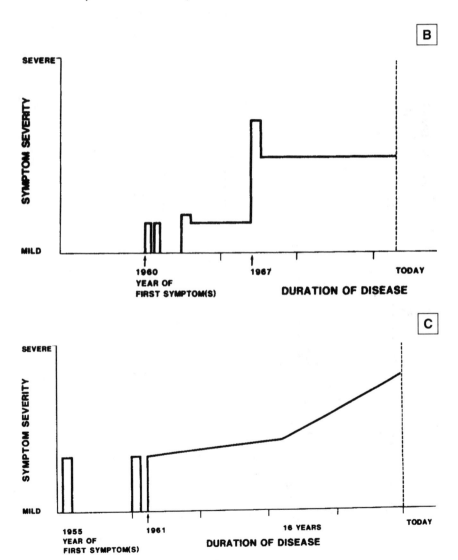

MEDICAL MANAGEMENT OF MULTIPLE SCLEROSIS

Medical management plans are developed based on the clinical course shown by each individual. Significant exacerbations are treated with high doses of cortisone products in an attempt to decrease the

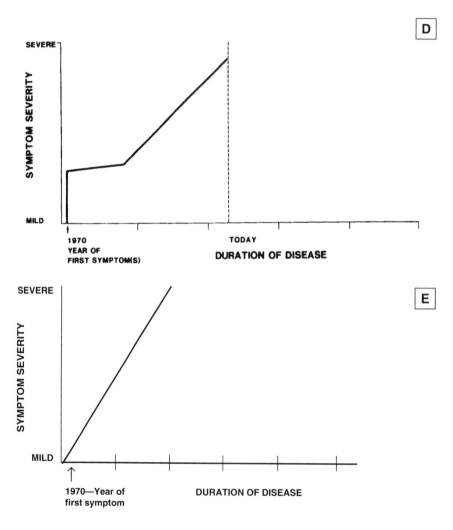

FIGURE 1.2 (CONTINUED)

edema associated with the acute immune, inflammatory response. With continued progression, the target of medical management becomes the immune system. Various immunosuppressant medications may be utilized to suppress the immune system. These are often the same medications used in transplant and cancer therapies.

No matter what the course of the MS, symptomatic therapy may be helpful. Symptoms are divided into three categories (Table 1.1):

1. Primary symptoms: these are caused directly by demyelination.
2. Secondary symptoms: these occur as the complications of primary symptoms.
3. Tertiary symptoms: these symptoms are the result of psychosocial dysfunction caused by MS.

Various medications and psychological strategies are recommended based on the above symptoms. Thus, despite the lack of a known cause, a number of therapeutic interventions aid in the management of MS.

Knowing that most MS is relatively benign, optimal management for nonprogressive MS revolves around education, appropriate exercise, and general good health habits. If the MS gives indication of progression, a more aggressive medical approach aimed at the immune system with immunosuppressant agents is often indicated.

TABLE 1.1 CATEGORIES OF SYMPTOMS IN MULTIPLE SCLEROSIS

1. Primary Symptoms	2. Secondary Symptoms
Weakness	Contractures
Numbness	Urinary tract infections
Visual disturbance	Decubiti
Dizziness	Pain
Ataxia	Cognitive
Bladder/bowel problems	
Sexual differences	3. Tertiary Symptoms
Pain	Psychological
Cognitive	Social

REHABILITATION PHILOSOPHY IN THE MANAGEMENT OF MULTIPLE SCLEROSIS

Many of the common symptoms and signs of MS are responsive to rehabilitation techniques. The rehabilitation of MS differs from that of medical conditions that are static, such as stroke, cerebral palsy, trauma, and from other progressive diseases such as the dystrophies and other inherited degenerative diseases. A major difference is the unpredictability of the disease both over its lifetime course and on a day-to-day basis. People with MS can feel strong one day and weak the next, or vice versa. While fatigue is not unique to MS, its variability is somewhat unusual (see Fatigue section in Chapter 3). Few diseases are as effected by affect; performance is much better when a patient is in good emotional health than when his/her mood is poor. The existence of multiple lesions within the CNS also complicates treatment, as each combination is unique to a given individual and produces a unique disease pattern.

The rehabilitation of MS is a constantly changing process because of the rapidity with which changes may occur. The therapist must therefore express confidence in the program but be capable of changing plans and goals on short notice. It is necessary to take a positive and realistic approach to a patient's changing problems.

A rehabilitation program should be recommended early in the course of the disease. Even when physical symptoms such as fatigue or visual problems are "invisible" to the therapist, rehabilitation can be very beneficial in improving the general condition of the patient and educating him/her about the disease and its management.

An appropriate rehabilitation program, no matter how extensive or how minimal, gives people a tremendous psychological boost because they are working to take charge of their own lives. This, coupled with the physical benefits that they can obtain, intensifies the importance of a good program. With a relatively mildly impaired individual, the role of the therapist may simply be one of educator, promoting good health, general conditioning, and recreation. With more moderate disease, a more aggressive approach must be introduced, such as introducing walking aids or providing assistance with activities of daily living (ADL). For a patient with more severe impairment, much more extensive adaptations may be required.

Many factors can complicate the rehabilitation of a patient with MS. Some relate to income, family structure, or living circumstances, while others involve specific effects of the disease on thought processes, which may manifest themselves as depression and/or problems in cognition.

Depression is common in MS, although it is certainly not unique to this disease. While its management is clearly beyond the scope of this book, it can substantially influence the outcome of rehabilitation. Depression is never cured by aggressive short-term rehabilitation. Longer, professional intervention is almost always essential, and depression must be appropriately managed before the rehabilitative process is begun. The rehabilitative and psychological professionals are clearly partners in the management of depression.

It is now well recognized that cognitive problems can and do occur in MS. Cognition involves memory, planning, foresight and judgment, and the ability to think clearly. For MS centers, cognitive deficits as a complicating factor in rehabilitation have become major issues, in large part because more complicated cases tend to cluster at such centers and their patients need more specialized help.

Cognitive problems in MS result from demyelination in the cerebral tracts that connect and integrate the primary sensory areas (visual, tactile, hearing, smell) to the motor, speech, and integration areas of the cerebrum. This results in poor recognition of deficits as well as an inability to store and retrieve new information, a combination which presents a major impediment to rehabilitation.

Often associated with these cognitive problems is a "pseudo" depression in which the individual may burst into tears or laughter inappropriately. This results from a lack of inhibition resulting from cerebral demyelination, and will also impede rehabilitation.

However, cognitive issues must be kept in perspective. While many people with MS have some cognitive problems, they are rarely severe enough to substantially impede rehabilitation. Some, a minority, have significant cognitive problems and will not be good candidates for rehabilitation. Unfortunately, beyond simplistic suggestions, such as substituting computers and pen and paper for decreased memory, there is at present no known effective rehabilitative approach for significant cognitive difficulties.

Despite such problems, the rehabilitative program is likely to be successful if each person with MS is assessed as an individual before assuming success or failure on the basis of his/her cognitive history. Pleasant surprises do occur.

RESTORATIVE REHABILITATION

The care of most chronic disabling diseases in our society is based on crisis intervention, with an emphasis on restoration of body functions. Restorative rehabilitation is therapy designed to enable an individual to attain the highest physical, emotional, and functional level possible within the constraints of a chronic disease. Traditionally, the focus of rehabilitation has been on individual muscle re-education and restoration, but when dealing with MS it must shift to a concern with the overall movement patterns of the patient, with specific consideration given to the key word "function."

Consideration must be given to self-care and ultimate functional gains. Self-care includes the ability to dress, bathe, eat, toilet, transfer, stair climb, and ambulate. It is important to look not only at movement patterns but at functional activities such as eating.

When assessing any treatment plan, the goals of the patient must be considered. Physical disability has a significant psychological impact in that it removes the sense of control over one's life. Control, defined in terms of realistic goals, must be placed within the patient's realm. This is often quite challenging, as many patients with MS may not have realistic goals about recovery and may experience many changes in their physical condition and performance abilities. For example, emphasis with the nonambulatory individual should be on wheelchair mobility, transfers, and self-care rather than on gait training. Programs should be highly individualized and also structured so that the patient clearly understands the treatment goals and what is and is not realistic. Goals also require a flexibility of expectations because the patient's condition often changes.

With restorative rehabilitation, specific goals are established and success can, to some extent, be determined by how successful the therapist is in bringing the patient to the completion of the goal. Thus when a patient's progress begins to plateau, a decision as to the effectiveness of the therapy must be made.

MAINTENANCE REHABILITATION

In contrast, the goal of maintenance rehabilitation is prevention of a decrease in function, whether directed toward a physical attribute as in muscle strength or toward emotional factors. Chronic diseases that have the potential to progress need ongoing attention in an attempt to help the patient to remain functionally stable in the face of a progressing neurological process. To deny people maintenance of their function is akin to voluntarily allowing their disease to progress.

Chronic progressive MS patients often exhaust all of their financial, supportive, and psychological resources in short order. Then, in desperation, early nursing home placement often follows. Formal professional maintenance rehabilitation establishes goals of both maintaining the individual physically and maintaining the family unit despite the presence of disabling disease. Its underlying hypothesis is that if an individual's capabilities can be maintained for a longer period of time, s/he may do better physically as well as psychologically.

Unfortunately, in the ever-changing health care of today, all too often insurance companies and governmental agencies dictate the care that will be provided to a given patient. Superficially, it can appear more economical to treat "maintenance" as unimportant. However, in the long run, this attitude will cost all of us far more dollars and result in far more disability. The establishment of maintenance programs for people with MS should be a primary focus of our health care system.

The maintenance program starts with a comprehensive initial evaluation, after which goals and treatment regimens are established. This is no different from more typical restorative programs. However, the emphasis is placed on goals and treatment to support and improve the present status. The program is specially designed for a person whose status has been declining and would in all likelihood continue to decline without rehabilitative services. With close observation, careful monitoring of changes in status can be made and early signs of potential problems addressed. Such preventative assessment is generally not feasible in most acute care restorative rehabilitation programs.

This type of ongoing rehabilitation is not inexpensive in terms of dollars, but its importance cannot be emphasized enough. Despite negative reinforcement from third-party payors, therapists must be cognizant of its usefulness.

IMPORTANCE OF DOCUMENTATION

A baseline therapy evaluation should be performed on most MS patients with any degree of disability. This objective data will help document the future course of the disease and permit realistic goals to be set. Because of the potential for rapid change in MS, re-evaluation may be necessary on a periodic basis. With these data, both the therapist and treating physician will be able to detect changes in medical status and determine the effectiveness of treatment.

The standard Subjective Objective Assessment Plan (SOAP) format is easily utilized to provide this information. The subjective information includes MS disease history, diagnostic information, current symptoms, prior therapy (physical/occupational/speech), psychosocial issues (living arrangements, current work status, transportation issues), ADL status, and levels of fatigue. Objective information includes evaluation and quantification of muscle tone, strength, joint range of motion, balance, coordination, pain, endurance, and dynamic activities including gait (with and without aids), one legged standing, etc. While doing the assessment, the following points are to be emphasized:

1. Any deficit in one motor area will affect the testing of the impairments. For example, increased muscle tone (spasticity) can influence true muscle testing, balance, range of motion, and gait.
2. Manual muscle testing requires accommodations dependent on the amount of spasticity. This may require various testing positions.
3. Muscle tone should be objectively measured (see Evaluation of Spasticity in Chapter 2)

4. Range of motion limitations may be due to soft tissue problems.

5. When testing balance and coordination, there must be an awareness of weakness, abnormal muscle tone, and postural problems. The quality of the movement must be observed.

6. During gait evaluation, attention must be placed on spasticity, weakness, balance, proprioception, and sensory loss.

7. Adaptive equipment evaluation must emphasize fit, efficiency, safety, and necessity.

8. Fatigue needs to be factored into the assessment.

A rehabilitation plan may then be formulated, with goals prioritized and formulated for each area assessed. The therapist, the patient, and the physician must then work together to formulate realistic goals.

2

PHYSICAL THERAPY

JULIE ARNDT, B.S., B.P.T., CHARLOTTE BHASIN, M.O.T., O.T.R./L.,
SURINDER P. BRAR, B.S., R.P.T., ROBERT HABASEVICH, M.S., R.P.T.,
JANIS JACOBS, M.S., L.P.T., KAREN TARBUCK-NELSON, B.S., R.P.T.,
RANDALL T. SCHAPIRO, M.D., ANDREA SELZER-SILVERMAN, O.T.R.,
AND JULIE VARNO, M.S., R.P.T.

SPASTICITY

Spasticity appears to be caused by a loss of normal modulating factors within the brain and spinal cord as the result of demyelination. It is a *velocity-dependent* response of passive stretch of a muscle which has three distinguishing characteristics: (1) the presence of a unidirectional hypertonicity, developed most fully in antigravity muscles; (2) an increase in this hypertonicity with increases in the velocity of muscle stretch; and (3) hyperactivity of the deep tendon reflexes. Normal muscle tone is influenced by the contractile state of the muscle, which, in turn, is determined partly by descending supraspinal signals impinging on the alpha motoneurons that innervate the peripheral musculature. With spasticity and the loss of the normal modulating neurons, passive motion of sufficient intensity and velocity results in an exaggerated resistance to the movement.

The presence of spasticity does not in itself justify its treatment, as spasticity does not always interfere with function. Abnormal muscle tone may in fact have some beneficial effects. When weakness in a muscle group is accompanied by a moderate amount of spasticity, the hypertonicity may allow for a more functional use of that muscle group. For example, a patient may be able to momentarily "stand on the spasticity" to accomplish transfers or even take a few steps with assistance; spasticity in the trunk may enhance sitting balance. However, significant spasticity causes movements to become inefficient and leads to increased fatigue. Balance may become impeded, causing poor gait patterns. Pain may result from the increased tone as well as the secondary abnormal gait patterns, and discomfort from spasms may be severely disabling. Subjectively the person with spasticity may complain of stiffness, pain, spasms, incoordination, weakness.

Evaluation of Spasticity

Many factors influence muscle tone, including fatigue, the weather, stress, body temperature, medications, and exercise. Despite these variables it is important to objectively assess spasticity prior to and following treatment. All the major muscle groups in the upper and lower extremities and the torso should be assessed.

There are several ways to objectify muscle tone. One method is passive movement performed by the therapist, with resistance to movement rated according to the Ashworth (and Modified Ashworth) Scale (Table 2.1). The Ashworth Scale ranges from 0 to 4; 0 indicates no increase in muscle tone and 4 indicates severe spasticity in flexion or extension. In this scale, grade 1 indicates a slight catch and release in flexion or extension, and 1+ is a slight increase in muscle tone, allowing minimal resistance during half the normal range of motion. Grade 2 is more marked increase in muscle tone through more than half the range of motion, but the affected part is easily moved. Grade 3 is considerable increase in muscle tone and passive movement is difficult. In grade four the affected part(s) is rigid in flexion or extension. As much as possible, each muscle group should be isolated to determine its tone.

Another method of tone assessment is to grade the patient using

TABLE 2.1 ASHWORTH MODIFIED SCALE OF MUSCLE TONE

GRADE 1	Slight catch and release in flexion and extension
GRADE 1+	Slight increase in muscle tone, allowing minimal response resisitance during half a range of motion
GRADE 2	More marked increase in muscle tone through most of range of motion
GRADE 3	Considerable increase in muscle tone; passive movement becomes difficult
GRADE 4	Affected part is rigid in flexion or extension

an ease of movement scale, where 0 is total ease and 10 is too stiff to move. The patient assigns a number to a specific movement before and immediately after treatment.

A *goniometer* can be used to measure active and/or passive movement pre- and post-treatment. Inferences can be made about muscle tone by observing and cataloguing the hierarchy of muscle function for the spastic muscle's antagonist pre- and post-treatment. Movement analysis of dynamic functional activity may be helpful, and video can be used to document functional movement before and after spasticity treatment. One must be aware that a supine or otherwise static test of spasticity in the lower extremities may not reveal the full extent of spasticity present during walking and other dynamic activities.

In general, the overall structure of every physical therapy treatment session should be to (1) test the physical function to be treated; (2) treat; (3) re-test the function. Spasticity responds differently depending on position, handling, movement, and inherent baseline level of central nervous system (CNS) excitability. The first task is to determine how to manage the spasticity so that it interferes least with function. For example, if the patient demonstrates hip extensor weakness and is unable to extend the hip in the prone position, it is counterproductive to assign prone hip extensor exercises. Rather, the therapist must determine a more appropriate position to work at alleviating the interfering spastic muscles. Patients who are unable to exercise in the prone or supine positions because of spasticity can improve their strength simply from exercising in the reflex-inhibiting, sidelying position.

Physical Management of Spasticity

Because the level of tension or relaxation has a significant effect on spasticity, a patient trying to decrease spasticity should be encouraged to be as relaxed as possible. A relaxed atmosphere can help, or a more formalized relaxation program such as visualization or biofeedback may be beneficial.

STRETCHING EXERCISES

Stretching exercises are highly beneficial in the management of spasticity (Figs. 2.1 and 2.2). Common muscle groups of the lower extremities that need emphasis from a stretching program include the hamstrings, adductors, gastroc-soleus groups, quadriceps, and the muscles of the ankle/foot. Using proper technique for stretching is important. Gentle sustained stretching is an effective way to decrease spasticity. It also helps to reduce circulatory stasis, prevent contractures, allow connective tissue and contractile elements to retain their appropriate relationship, provide added sensory stimulation by activating proprioceptors and mechanoreceptors, and helps reset alpha and gamma muscle spindles for adjusting tone.

The stretch should be held at the point where the patient just starts to feel discomfort, and s/he should be reminded not to go beyond this level. It is most effective when 1–2 minutes is spent in the stretch position at a point where a gentle pulling sensation is felt, without stretching into the painful range. A gentle pressure should be applied to "take up the slack" as the spasticity decreases and the muscles gently stretch. The key is to allow the muscles to elongate through relaxation, not to overcome the inherent elasticity and resistance offered by the connective tissue and contractile elements. This same result can be obtained by stretches the patient can be taught to do him/herself, passive stretches taught to significant others, or by the use of a positioning slant board (Fig. 2.3). Stretching should not

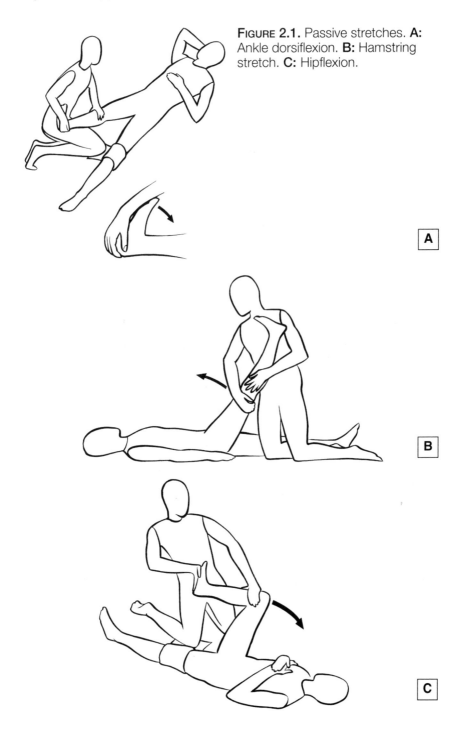

FIGURE 2.1. Passive stretches. **A:** Ankle dorsiflexion. **B:** Hamstring stretch. **C:** Hipflexion.

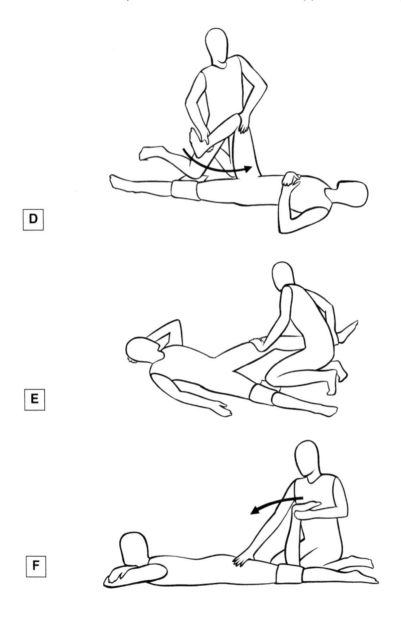

FIGURE 2.1 (CONTINUED). Passive stretches. D: Internal-external rotation. E: Abduction-adduction. F: Knee flexing.

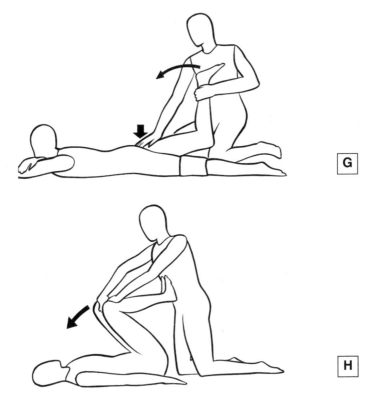

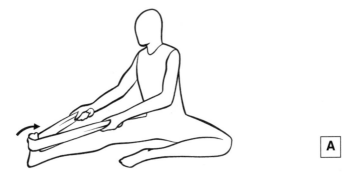

FIGURE 2.1 (CONTINUED). Passive stretches. **G:** Hip extension. **H:** Trunk flexion.

FIGURE 2.2. Independent stretches. **A:** Heel cord.

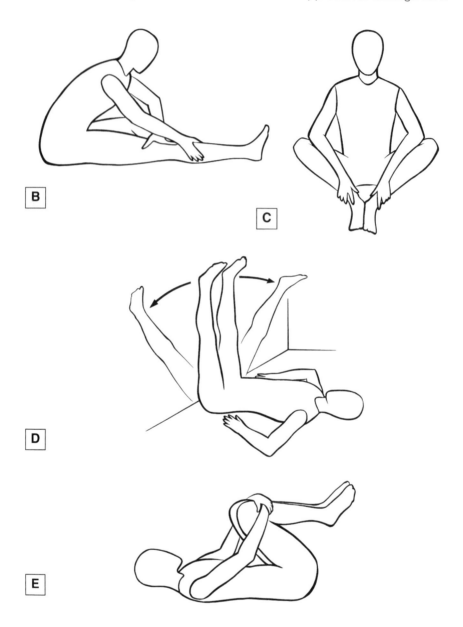

FIGURE 2.2 (CONTINUED). Independent stretches. B: Hamstring. C: Butterfly sit. D: Wall stretch. E: Knee hug.

produce muscle spasms. Teach the patient the proper positioning for each stretch, e.g., for stretching the hamstrings, the movement occurs between the femur and the pelvis. Stretching exercises should be performed at least once daily for the best results, and should be performed before other exercise routines to enhance the positive effects.

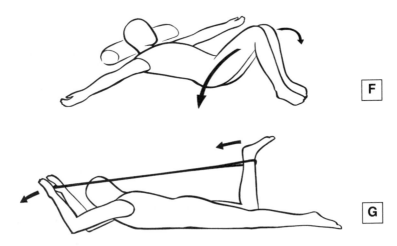

FIGURE 2.2 (CONTINUED). Independent stretches. F: Hook lying. G: Belt pull.

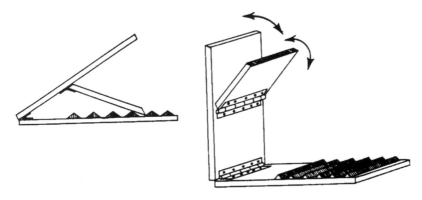

FIGURE 2.3. Positioning slant board may aid in stretching.

SUMMARY A stretching routine should allow elongation of the muscles through relaxation, not by overcoming the inherent elasticity and resistance offered by the connective tissue and contractile elements. The stretch should not produce muscle spasm, and neither the patient nor the therapist should ever perform rapid movements into the stretch range.

MOVEMENT PATTERNS

Reflex-inhibiting movement patterns not only inhibit abnormal postural reactions, but also facilitate active automatic and voluntary movements. Facilitation is accomplished using "key points of control" (Fig. 2.4). The main key points are proximally at the head and spine, shoulder and pelvic girdles; and distally at the toes and ankles, fingers and wrist. Simultaneously exercising several such control points can be extremely beneficial. These include the *head, arms and shoulder girdle, and legs and pelvis.*

HEAD Extension of the head combined with extension of the shoulder girdle in the prone-lying, sitting, or standing position inhibits flexor spasticity and facilitates extension in the rest of the body. Simultaneous flexion of the head and the shoulder girdle inhibits extensor spasticity or spasms.

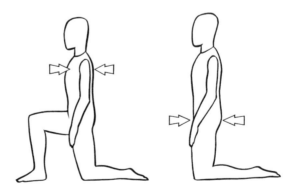

Figure 2.4. Some key points of motor control.

ARMS AND SHOULDER GIRDLE   Horizontal abduction of the arms in external rotation combined with supination and extended elbows inhibits flexor spasticity, especially of the pectorals, and facilitates spontaneous opening of the hand and fingers. Elevation of the arms in outward rotation inhibits flexor spasticity, and downward pressure of the arms and shoulder girdle helps extension of the spine. Abduction of the thumb with a supinated arm, and extended wrist if possible, facilitates opening of all the fingers.

LEGS AND PELVIS   Flexion of the hips facilitates abduction, external rotation, and ankle dorsiflexion and inhibits leg extensor spasticity. Abduction of the legs is also facilitatory with external rotation and extension. External rotation in extension facilitates abduction and dorsiflexion of the ankles. Dorsiflexion of the toes, especially the outer three or four, inhibits extensor spasticity throughout the leg and facilitates dorsiflexion of the ankle, and external rotation and abduction of the leg.

POSITIONING   Positioning also significantly affects movement patterns. There are four basic positions in which the exercises can be performed: prone, supine, sitting, and side-lying.(Fig. 2.5):

PRONE: Extension of the hips and legs is facilitated by raising the head with the arms extended above the head and the spine extended. However, this stretch is not beneficial when extensor spasticity of the legs is present. If this position is combined with horizontal abduction of the arms, it will facilitate extension of the dorsal spine, opening of the fingers, and abduction of the legs (Fig. 2.5A).

SUPINE: Abduction with external rotation and extension of the hips and knees will inhibit both flexor and extensor spasticity in the legs. Still further reduction can be obtained by also dorsiflexing the toes and ankle and abduction of the great toe (Fig. 2.5B).

SITTING: Flexion of the hips, trunk well forward, legs abducted, all facilitate extension of the spine and raising the head (Fig. 2.5C).

SIDELYING: The sidelying position often normalizes tone when supported in a neutral position with the topside more inhibited than the bottom (Fig. 2.5D).

SUMMARY: Positioning helps to decrease spasticity by inhibiting primitive reflex patterns that do not allow normal movements. In general,

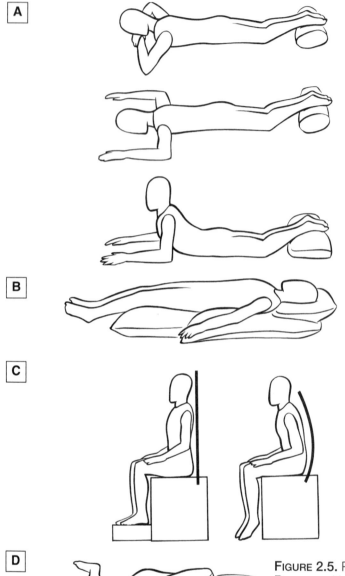

FIGURE 2.5. Positioning. **A:** Prone position for stretching. **B:** Supine position for stretching. **C:** Sitting position (**left:** correct; **right:** incorrect). **D:** Sidelying position.

the supine position facilitates extensor tone and inhibits flexor tone; the prone position facilitates flexor tone and inhibits extensor tone.

MOVEMENT TECHNIQUES

Various movement techniques can be used to modulate spasticity and allow the patient to experience the sense of normal movement and normal posture. The earlier treatment is initiated, the more likely the patient is to retain normal movement. The following techniques are useful in attempting to attain normal movement:

1. Rhythmic passive and assisted active trunk rotation.
2. Systematic rolling, as from supine to sidelying, may decrease spasticity. As the patient is rolled away, the greatest inhibition is to the extremities on the top. Adding shoulder girdle or pelvic/trunk rotation will assist in decreasing spasticity. Rhythmical rotation of an individual extremity can also be helpful. The limb is supported and rotated alternately in both directions in a slow, rhythmical manner around a longitudinal axis for approximately 10 seconds. Once relaxation is achieved, the limb is moved actively or passively into the newly gained range.
3. Slow, rhythmical rocking can be done in any of the developmental patterns/positions. It is easily combined with other techniques, such as in quadruped over a ball, which combines inversion and weight bearing with slow rocking.

SLOW STROKING/PRESSURE TECHNIQUES

Slow stroking may decrease overall muscle tone and allow the muscles to relax. For paraspinal muscle treatment, the patient is usually prone or hooklying with the back exposed. A light but firm pressure is applied as the therapist uses the flat of the hand to stroke the paravertebral muscles from T-1 to L-2, moving about 2 inches per second. As the moving hand reaches the lumbar area, the second hand makes contact at T-1 and begins to stroke, making certain that the top hand is placed before removing the bottom hand. This should only be done for approximately 3–5 minutes, or it tends to become facilitatory.

A firm maintained pressure applied to the upper lip, palms of the hand, soles or sides of the feet, or abdominal area can produce a generalized decrease in spasticity. The maintained pressure can be applied directly by the therapist, or by positioning the patient so his/her own body weight provides the necessary pressure.

Firm pressure on the muscle's point of insertion can be used to produce relaxation. Pressure can be applied manually or by using a supportive surface. This technique is very useful in obtaining greater range of motion in patients with moderate to severe spasticity and can be easily incorporated into a range of motion (ROM) program.

FUNCTIONAL ELECTRIC STIMULATION

Functional electric stimulation (FES) provides spasticity relief in many patients with grade 1–2 mild-to-moderate spasticity, especially those with mild spasticity in a relatively small number of muscle groups. However, FES may improve a nonambulatory patient's ability to control the lower extremities and torso during transfers, and can release hip adductor spasticity, permitting improved self-care. The electrodes are placed over the belly of the muscle with the negative electrode over the point which elicits the strongest palpable or visual muscle contraction. The intensity should be within the patient's tolerance and should not produce discomfort. In order to obtain a therapeutic result, the stimulus should produce at least a palpable muscle contraction; more desirably, it should produce a visible muscle contraction and possibly a joint movement. After the optimal treatment frequency and protocol are determined, the patient can be treated in a physical therapy clinic or provided with a home FES unit.

COLD PACKS

The application of ice packs or ice massage may be helpful in reducing tone. There are two common methods. One is to immerse a towel into a bucket of slush, wring it out, and apply it directly to the spastic muscle. The towel is changed every several minutes, for a total of 5–20 minutes. Alternately, the spastic hand or foot can be immersed in a container of ice water. This may be rather stressful, and is contraindicated if the patient has poor circulation or considers the treatment too noxious or painful.

MEDICATIONS

Medications may also be used to decrease muscle tone. A number of medications are available, all of which require experience to utilize effectively. These include baclofen (Lioresal), diazepam (Valium), dantrolene (Dantrium), cyclobenzaprine (Flexoril), clonazapam (Klonopin), and carbamazepine (Tegretol). The most widely used drug for managing spasticity in multiple sclerosis (MS) is baclofen, whose site of action is the spinal cord. Total dosages range from 5 mg to over 100 mg per day, and titration of the dose is essential. A small starting dose is gradually increased over a period of weeks until a therapeutic dose is achieved. Side effects are usually minimal, but include drowsiness and weakness. Too high a dose results in too little tone in the legs to sustain an erect posture.

Diazapam and clonazapam, whose site of action is the brain, have significant drawbacks of being heavily sedating and of producing chemical dependancy. They have a rapid onset of action and are very effective for nocturnal spasms. Dantrolene acts directly on the muscle. Often, dantrolene administration produces weakness in MS patients, and judicious use is essential. Low doses may serve as an adjunct to the other, better-tolerated medications. Carbamazepine, an anticonvulsant, often aids in managing spasms associated with too much muscle tone. Sedation is a common side effect, and the white blood cell count must be observed. Cyclobenzaprine is used for back pain and accompanying spasms. However, it also has an effect on spasticity and may be used accordingly.

Only physicians may prescribe these medications but it is essential for the therapist to communicate the effect of the medication on the patient's spasticity to the treating physician, to allow for a coordinated and full therapeutic approach.

BALANCE AND COORDINATION

Impairment of balance and/or coordination in MS may be the result of abnormalities almost anywhere within the CNS. The cerebellum is frequently involved and balance problems are therefore quite common. Cerebellar disease may result in ataxia with incoordination of any or all of the extremities, or in an intention tremor that becomes exaggerated with movement. Lesions of the brainstem may result in exactly the same symptoms, since the outflow tracts of the cerebellum flow through the brainstem.

The posterior columns transmit sensory input from the extremities to the brain. Since position sense is crucial to balance, demyelination of the posterior columns results in balance problems. These tracts travel great distances in the spinal cord, and are therefore readily impaired by lesions at a variety of neurologic levels.

The optic nerves are frequently demyelinated, and the absence of appropriate visual input can affect balance. Decreased visual acuity may cause balance problems, but skewed or double vision is more frequently the cause of a balance problem.

The parietal lobes organize a high percentage of sensory input, and abnormalities in these areas result in abnormal input. This often occurs at a level below consciousness, and the patient may therefore not be aware of his/her poor balance, making rehabilitation more difficult. In addition, weakness and spasticity are often complicating variables in managing balance and coordination problems.

Assessment of Coordination

Coordination involves many elements of movement control. As much as is feasible, each element should be tested separately. Target hitting with the index finger and the big toe can be used to measure accuracy of movement and to assess movement control in space. Appropriate control of movement in space includes the ability to control direction, quality, and speed. The presence and degree of tremor can be documented, and even grossly estimated in inches or centimeters. Control of speed of movement can be assessed by observing the patient deliver a blow with both upper extremities and stamping the floor with the plantar surface of each foot separately. In analyzing speed of movement, one should assess and document speed control, direction control, accuracy, cushioning control at impact, and movement reversal control.

Coordination involves a sequence of muscle action. One way to assess alternate agonist/antagonist coordination at the ankle is to have the patient tap his/her foot while in a sitting position, with the hip at 90 degrees and the knee flexed to approximately 70 degrees. In assessing coordination during foot tapping it is useful to observe it at slow, medium and fast speeds. In the presence of spasticity or other causes of incoordination, decompensation of movement may be observed only during the faster speed activities.

Upper extremity coordination and sequencing of muscle action can be assessed by observing alternate/reciprocal movement of the forearm pronators and supinators and/or the wrist flexors and extensors. Coordination of the wrist flexors and extensors can be observed by having the patient perform a rapid and relaxed wave of the hand, with the movement occurring at the wrist, which involves proper sequencing of wrist flexors and extensors.

The patient's motor planning and preparatory posture for movement and activity should be carefully assessed, noting whether s/he prepares for a movement or whether s/he engages in a movement or activity without proper forethought and body positioning for its success. Preparatory posture can be assessed during the entire evaluation, as the patient is asked to perform various maneuvers.

Timing the onset of a movement can be done using a moving target. The examiner may move the finger in a prearranged, predictable pattern and the patient is asked to tap the examiner's finger in the middle of the movement range, and return to the starting position. The therapist should note the appropriateness of the timing of the onset of the motion, including whether the task was completed accurately, with fluid motion and without compensatory maneuvers.

In performing maneuvers requiring coordination, the therapist should note interference of spasticity with voluntary movement including reflex patterns, compensatory muscle contractions, and involuntary or compensatory movement for both limbs and torso. Such reflex patterns and compensatory movements should be correlated with the attempted voluntary motion during which they occur.

Assessment of Balance

Balance also involves many elements of movement control. Standing balance is assessed initially with the patient standing comfortably without assistive device. Progressively, the pedestal base (distance between the feet) is narrowed until the feet are together, heels and toes. In the narrowest position that can be accomplished, the patient is asked to close the eyes while the examiner pushes gently at the shoulders to create a momentary imbalance (Romberg test). This may then be repeated with one foot in front of the other (tandem position).

Sitting balance is assessed by asking the patient to assume a sitting position while the examiner observes trunkal stability during stimulatory pushes at the shoulder and trunk.

Kneeling balance is assessed in a similar fashion with the patient kneeling. Lifting one extremity off the surface may add information to the evaluation. Alternating arm and leg movement may be helpful.

Some positions which may aid in the testing and rehabilitation of balance problems are illustrated in Figure 2.6.

Therapeutic Management of Balance and Coordination

When working on balance activities it is important to work from low to high center of gravity, from static to dynamic activities, and from wide to narrow base of support. The activities should be challenging but not too difficult for the patient, or little relearning will occur. In addition, attempting stressful activities may increase spasticity, which probably will decrease balance abilities. It is often beneficial to combine balance activities with slow rocking or weight shift to decrease spasticity, and then progress to higher level skills.

A visual cue that has proven helpful to improve balance is to have the patient focus on an object at eye level approximately 20–30 feet in front of him/her, and then to readjust as the distance decreases to 10–15 feet.

Developmental sequence positions can help to improve balance in functional positions. The same sequence of positions is recommended, progressing from a wide base, low center of gravity to more mature positions. The therapist must separate, to some extent, weakness from balance problems, and weakness and spasticity should be treated before balance.

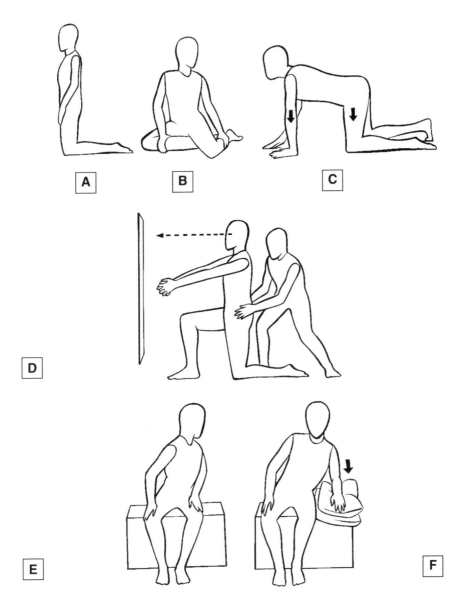

FIGURE 2.6. Balance and coordination. A: Kneeling. B: Sitting. C: 4-Point kneeling. Note equal distribution of weight over the 4 points of contact. D: Stand kneeling. This position develops increased balance by establishing pelvic and hip control. E: Turning to look behind. This exercise challenges the balance system. F: Taking weight through affected arm.

RETRAINING BALANCE

Patients have often developed soft tissue shortening to such an extent that they are unable to move the pelvis into sufficient anterior tilt to reach the neutral alignment position. Normal balance control requires that the pelvis move freely enough to allow lumbar extension while maintaining the upper thorax in an absolutely upright position. Shortened soft tissue must be treated prior to initiating voluntary positional control exercises, and range of motion must be improved to enable the patient to assume the required positions. Positioning techniques can be used to prepare the patient with hip extensor spasticity for balance control work. For example, the patient may be brought into flexion at the hip joint, with the torso flexed forward, before s/he can maintain an upright position. The motion occurs between the pelvis and the femur, so that the torso is almost laying on the thighs. This maneuver is helpful in decreasing hip extensor spasticity, and may allow the pelvis to move into a neutral position while sitting upright.

The first step in sitting balance retraining is to relearn the neutral position of the torso and pelvis in relation to the thorax, and the entire torso in relation to the ground. Tactile, verbal, and visual cues can be used to reteach the upright position to the patient. These same techniques can be utilized in retraining positional control of the thorax with respect to the pelvis. The easiest maneuver for the patient to perform is "placing." The therapist uses manual or tactile techniques to place the pelvis into a neutral position, with the thorax centered over the pelvis. The patient then attempts to hold the thorax and pelvis in this position, or "place." At first, the patient may need assistance to perform the maneuver. If s/he has sufficient muscle strength, the learning process for positional control should take one to two weeks. It may be necessary to specifically teach pelvic control and to use the supine position for each pelvic movement through the entire range from extreme anterior pelvic tilt to extreme posterior pelvic tilt.

When this maneuver has been mastered in the supine position with knees flexed, the patient can progress to the supine position with the legs extended, then to sitting or standing, whichever position the therapist is using in the balance retraining. As soon as the patient is aware and able to control pelvic movement and positioning, the essence of balance retraining is much easier to grasp. When s/he can maintain upper body neutral position, unsupported, then s/he progresses to movement from an off-center position to moving into the neutral position alignment in sitting. Working from several off-center starting positions is important: a torso forward-flexed position, a torso side-flexed position, both right and left, a diagonal position from rear-side, both right and left, and from a position of the torso posterior to midline. The easiest way to perform this maneuver is to move the entire torso, as a unit, from off-center to neutral.

If the patient is unable to perform an anterior-posterior tilt maneuver, this must be taught. The pelvic tilt is best taught initially in a supine position with the knees flexed and feet flat on the ground. Each individual responds differently to verbal and spatial cues. After mastering this pelvic movement in the supine position with the knees flexed, the patient should practice the pelvic tilt with hips and knees extended to neutral (in the supine position), progressing to holding and maintaining the pelvic tilt while one knee is flexed to the chest and returned to neutral position, without allowing the pelvic tilt to release. The progression is to performing the pelvic tilt in the standing position, while leaning the torso against the wall. During this maneuver, the feet should be placed approximately 6" out from the wall. After mastering this sequence of maneuvers, the patient is ready to perform the pelvic tilt in the standing position. At this point, if s/he is able to perform the maneuver through full range of pelvic motion, it is appropriate to begin other alignment control awareness instruction and practice.

The process of attending to each alignment component should be incorporated into one exercise period. The patient should practice this daily. The expected progression is to move into the new neutral alignment positioning very rapidly without having to attend to each component. This may take several days to several weeks to learn. After this is mastered, the patient is encouraged to move from the off-center position to neutral while simultaneously moving the pelvis and thorax into neutral.

GENERAL TECHNIQUES

The therapist can make use of the following techniques in attempting to improve balance.

JOINT APPROXIMATION TECHNIQUES When applied in the direction of weight bearing, these techniques allow for co-contraction of muscles around the weight-bearing joints, increasing stability.

ALTERNATIVE SENSORY FEEDBACK The eyes may be used to facilitate appropriate movements if vibratory or proprioceptive input has been lost.

BIOFEEDBACK AND RELAXATION TRAINING Employing these techniques may decrease tremors of the head, hand, and trunkal ataxia, allowing the patient to perform simple ADL skills.

PRACTICING THE COMPONENT PARTS OF AN ACTIVITY Balance in one specific functional activity can often be achieved by breaking down the activity into its component parts. As an example, sitting can be achieved through the following steps: Have the patient assume a neutral body position alignment. Develop sufficient pelvic mobility using anterior and posterior tilting to permit movement at the trunk. Develop sufficient range of motion at the trunk and hips to assume a good sitting posture. Verbal, tactile, and visual cues can be used to train the patient in an appropriate sitting posture. Mirrors may be helpful. The movement through states of sitting must be slowly progressive, but when mastered, further progression to off-center trunk positions may occur. Once those skills are mastered, progression to using the upper extremities while maintaining good independent sitting posture, i.e., catching a ball, may be possible.

HIGHER LEVEL BALANCE ACTIVITIES

The therapist can make use of balance boards, balance beams, and Swiss balls and computerized equipment such as the Balance Master. To improve higher level balance activities such as hopping on one foot, tandem walking and running are helpful. The patient may also be challenged with other exercises, e.g., riding a bicycle, skiing, playing tennis. The therapist needs to reinforce the theory of continuing practice in order to improve some of the higher level skills.

Plasticity and Compensation Techniques

The term "plasticity" refers to the ability of one part of the CNS to take over the function of another. While theoretically possible, it rarely occurs in the adult brain and spinal cord. It is therefore not practical to design a rehabilitation program that utilizes plasticity. In children, the process appears much more practical and has numerous advantages. The rehabilitation of balance and coordination abnormalities is therefore primarily geared to techniques that teach the patient compensation techniques to improve his/her response to balance challenges. This may involve using adaptive equipment to improve ADL skills. For example, arm and wrist weights may make eating easier by decreasing the tremors in the hand and arm, weighted canes may provide more stability for those with ataxia of the lower extremities, and a button hook may make the fine coordinated activity of buttoning much easier.

At times, patients may be reluctant to try aids or adaptive equipment because they feel that independence is being lost. It is crucial for the therapist to explain and clarify the positive benefits of adaptive aids. At the same time, compliance will be much better if the therapist listens to the patient and provides some choices. Many patients with tremor welcome adaptive aids as a way to communicate to others the presence of a physical handicap.

Cognitive Aspects of Motor Training

Recent learning theory emphasizes the importance of the cognitive learning process in motor retraining. This involves using every method possible to provide the patient with increasing awareness about his/her body position and movement and options for motor control. The therapist's use of movement and positioning, of mirrors, and of tactile and manual cues, may be very effective in improving the patient's understanding of his/her present level of function and the level desired. In addition, many patients effectively use imagery to improve movement or positional control. Some may need specific instruction in how to image and exactly which images may be most effective. One effective technique is to teach the exact maneuver until the patient has a very clear understanding of the desired movement. Then s/he images performing the desired movement in a fluid, controlled manner. As soon as s/he has completed the image, s/he then moves the body into the image, which is already performing this smooth movement or the positional maneuver with ease.

Patients with severe cognitive problems may be unable to benefit from such techniques, but the majority will find them useful.

STRENGTH

Weakness is a common problem in MS and has numerous and varied causes. Obviously, demyelination of the long pyramidal tracts can cause an upper motoneuron type of weakness, apparently related to a decreased or complete block of conduction.

Spasticity often results from demyelination, and can simulate weakness by increasing the activity in the antagonistic muscle groups. Not only does the muscle have to move the limb against gravity, but also against the resistance caused by the spasticity opposing its motion.

Fatigue can also cause apparent weakness. The fatigue may be local, involving poor neural conduction to the muscle, or it may be a general result of decreased functional strength.

Apraxia, or the inability to perform a skilled act despite the preservation of the motor components involved in the act, may mimick weakness. This symptom may result from demyelination of the parietal lobe or along the posterior columns.

Impaired sensation, especially decreased proprioception, may limit the person with MS by preventing the "fine tuning" of movement. This decreases efficiency significantly, producing weakness.

Disuse due to decreased activity level is another etiology for weakness in MS. Decreased activity is often due to more challenged mobility, decreased tolerance to activity, or decreased desire for activity due to depression.

Designing a Strengthening Program

When designing a successful strengthening program, the therapist must consider several questions: (1) How extensive is the weakness? (2) How long has it been present? (3) What is its specific etiology (type)? The tendency of most therapists when they see weakness is to consider weight training. In MS this often has a very poor result. When weakness is due to demyelination in the pyramidal tracts (MS plaques), progressively resistant muscle-strengthening exercises will only increase fatigue and thus increase weakness. It is extremely important to analyze the patient's condition carefully in order to determine appropriate treatment.

Muscle Testing

A conventional muscle test should be performed if there is no abnormal muscle tone and functional strength assessment should be made for all muscles, even if abnormal tone is present. When testing strength in the presence of abnormal muscle tone, the therapist should use special positioning and handling techniques, noting the configuration of the weakness. It is important to be aware that the sidelying position is the preferred one for decreasing spasticity in hip muscle groups. If spasticity is present in the plantar flexors, the ankle dorsiflexors will perform differently when the knee is flexed or extended. These factors should be taken into consideration during the evaluation.

Documentation of the results of muscle-strength testing is imperative. The conventional muscle test documentation is a scale from 0 to 5: 0 is a muscle with no movement, not even a twitch; 1 is a muscle which can twitch but otherwise not move; 2 is a muscle that can move but not withstand the force of gravity; 3 is a muscle that can withstand gravity but no added resistance; 4 is a muscle which is stronger than gravity but not normal; and 5 is a strong muscle. The amount of resistance should be documented when muscle tone is abnormal. A verbal scale, e.g., good, fair, poor, can be used if the test position is noted along with how much voluntary movement is present through the available range of motion. In any strength documentation, the passive range of motion at all joints should also be evaluated and joint integrity should be assessed.

General Principles of a Strengthening Program

Following are common principles to remember while implementing a strengthening program.

1. Unaffected muscle groups should be maximally strengthened to allow maximal use of compensation techniques that involve unaffected limbs.

2. Use adaptive devices, i.e., canes and crutches, to allow the patient to remain ambulatory longer and maintain functional strength levels as long as possible.

3. Strengthening exercises must be safe and efficacious. Therapists must teach the patient a judicious balance between rest and exercise.

4. The patient should progress through the strengthening program very slowly. For example, if s/he is starting at 8–10 repetition (reps) of each exercise, s/he can increase 1–2 reps every 2–3 weeks, to 20–25 reps. One- to two-pound weights may then be added and the reps decreased to 8-10, with the progression starting over. This slow increase in progression accompanied by good compliance will lead to successful strengthening. A cool atmosphere allows for more efficient exercise, as MS patients are often highly sensitive to heat.

5. Home programs for these exercises are essential; the effectiveness of any exercise program depends on its being carried out on an ongoing basis.

6. Prior to strengthening, stretching exercises should be performed to decrease spasticity, increase flexibility, and increase blood flow to the area.

7. To improve functional strength, exercises should be performed at submaximal resistance with frequent repetitions.

8. Emphasis should be placed on proximal strengthening in order to decrease energy consumption during functional activities.

9. Large fluid movements to enhance coordination should be used.

10. If a patient has difficulty initiating movement, try starting with large body/trunk movements, then moving from proximal to distal.

11. Light weights may help stabilization if a patient has significant tremors.

12. Combining strengthening exercises with aerobic, balance, and/or spasticity-reducing exercises whenever possible will maximize benefits within the patient's exercise tolerance.

13. Avoid excessive fatigue of a muscle: 1–5-minute rest periods throughout the exercise session will facilitate recovery of neurotransmission.

14. Set realistic goals and expectations with the patient. Be creative, realistic, and simplistic. The more enjoyable the exercises, the better the compliance.

Examples of routine strengthening positions are illustrated in Figure 2.7

AMBULATION

Decreased ability to walk is one of the more common rehabilitation problems in MS. Gait is involved for a number of reasons, including muscle weakness, spasticity, impaired sensation and proprioception, balance disturbances, rapid onset of fatigue, visual problems, vertigo, and apraxia.

The analysis and treatment of complicated gait problems requires careful observation, discussion of the issues with the patient, and the setting of realistic goals in participation with the patient. Ambulation is extremely important to patients with MS, and the therapist should offer some perspective to keep its relative importance in proportion. The patient should be encouraged to realize that ambulation is not necessarily a measurement of independence, nor should it be allowed to define ones physical image of being healthy.

Treatment of Ambulation Problems
TRUNK CONTROL

The principles of achieving trunk control are discussed above in the section on balance. Good trunk control is essential to improving gait and should be attained before other interventions are begun.

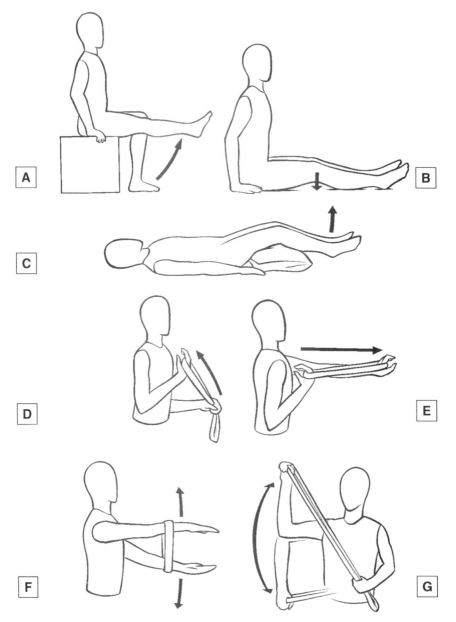

FIGURE 2.7. Strengthening exercises. A: Knee extension. B: Quad set. C: Terminal knee extension. D: Elbow flexion with Theraband. E: Elbow extension with Theraband. F: Shoulder flexion-extension with Theraband.

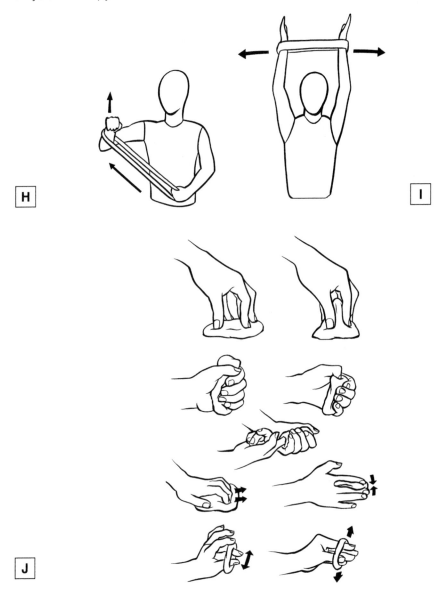

G: External rotation with Theraband. **H:** Shoulder abduction with Theraband. **I:** Shoulder adduction with Theraband. **J:** Exercises for strengthening fingers with use of putty.

Once this is accomplished, the stage is set for higher progressive stages in ambulation to be worked on.

FLEXIBILITY

Improving flexibility in the trunk, pelvis, and in the major muscle groups of the lower extremities is also important in improving or restoring normal gait. Additionally, the use of inhibiting techniques for spasticity (see above section Physical Management of Spasticity) will allow better motor control at the joints of the lower extremities. If flexibility is improved and spasticity is well managed, the patient will not have to use as much energy or strength to initiate or complete movements during walking.

STRENGTH

Gait is often more functional when strength can be improved in the trunk and lower extremities (see above section Strength). Muscle groups that tend to weaken earliest in MS include the hip flexors, hip abductors, dorsiflexors, and ankle evertors and invertors. Compensatory strengthening programs should be started when weakness is first detected. Because it is physically difficult if not impossible to strengthen a muscle whose weakness is the result of central demyelination, the therapist must often be creative to help the patient.

BALANCE

Improving balance in the various positions of the developmental sequence will also enhance gait training. In order to maintain good, safe, independent gait, the therapist should utilize higher level balance training techniques, e.g., one leg standing balance, hopping, and tandem walking. Further discussion of this is found above in the section on balance. The therapist moves the patient through progressive stages of standing balance, beginning with good independent static balance, moving to independent dynamic balance (weight-shifting activities), and progressing to functional activities in standing. Finally, the move is to one-leg standing activities. With these balance training movements, the therapist can teach the patient to use more appropriate ankle balance strategies, when indicated, rather than hip strategies. Patients with minimal balance problems often improve noticeably with an intense balance training program, and those with moderate-to-severe balance problems can frequently see some improvement in specific areas within months of consistent therapy 1–2 times per week.

ENDURANCE

Improving endurance in walking is also of the utmost importance, because fatigue is a common problem that limits functional gait. The therapist should teach moderation of gait activities, utilizing rest periods with a slow progressive scale of increasing distance over a period of 2–4 weeks. For example, if a patient can walk only a block before fatiguing, the therapist would suggest walking one block three to four times per week for about 2–3 weeks, then increase the distance from one block to 1½ or 2 blocks for 2–3 weeks at three to four times per week. With this slow progression, the patient will both feel successful and improve endurance. The patient must remember the importance of consistency and become aware of body cues to avoid excessive fatigue.

BODY AWARENESS

The use of visual and tactile cues that enhance better posture can be helpful in improving gait. Mirrors and appropriate sensory feedback may enhance motor control during the various phases of the gait pattern. The therapist can stimulate the patient to develop a smoother gait pattern by using various facilitation techniques to enhance adequate hip flexion during the initial swing phase and by encouraging dorsiflexion during this phase. Helping the patient to develop body awareness of the results of compensatory techniques and of any abnormal posture during gait may also improve the gait pattern.

Ambulation Aids

In order to remain walking as long as possible the process must be extremely efficient. Ambulation aids thus become an important consideration. With the proper use of the appropriate aid, the patient can improve safety, decrease energy cost, and increase endurance while ambulating. However, the issue of assistive devices raises complicated emotional issues for many people with MS. The MS person often resists aids because they are perceived as symbols of disability and dependence. The therapist should provide helpful information to identify and address these emotional issues. The goal is for the person to improve function, and whatever tools it takes to accomplish this are essential. The aids themselves should be viewed much as a carpenter views his/her tools—they are inanimate and nonemotional. The patient needs the best tools available and must learn how to use them; the therapist can guide the patient in diluting the emotional issues associated with the aids.

Often the patient needs good upper extremity function to use an aid effectively and safely. Significant cerebellar disease or weakness will therefore impede the use of the ambulation aid, and patients with severe visual or cognitive problems may not be able to use assistive devices safely.

The most commonly used ambulatory aids are one cane, two canes, light-weight forearm crutches, quad cane, ankle-foot orthoses (AFO), and walkers (Fig. 2.8). The therapist's knowledge of assistive devices and of the patient's current walking ability based on evaluation of gait are essential in determining when a patient needs a walking aid and which one will be most helpful. The therapist must properly fit the aid to the patient and teach the appropriate method for its optimal use. One cane is usually sufficient to compensate for minimal balance problems. If the problems are more severe or if one cane does not provide enough support, bilateral supports such as light-weight forearm crutches or even a walker should be recommended. The therapist will need to carefully evaluate specific problems such as weakness, spasticity, ataxia, and fatigue. The patient's upper extremity motor control and his/her control over the trunk and lower extremities are also important. The proper recommendation of assistive devices accompanied by proper training will allow patients to remain ambulatory longer. Some patients may be ambulatory with aids only for short distances, or only in the mornings, but may need other mobility assistance such as wheelchairs or electric carts for longer distances and for afternoons. Even such short distance ambulation should be encouraged. Maintaining this functional level can provide much independence in ADL skills and help the patient to maintain independence.

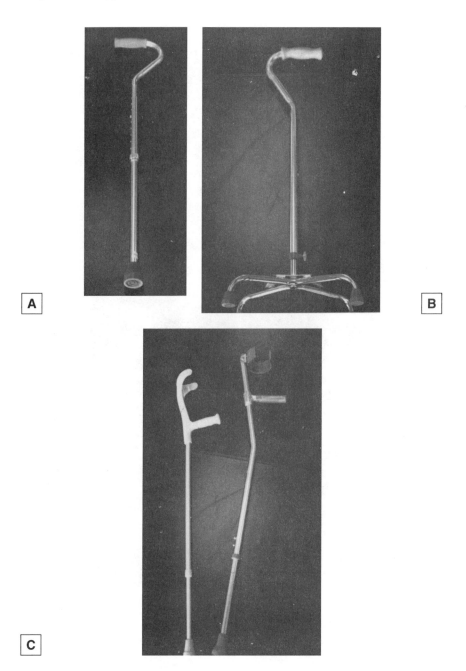

FIGURE 2.8. Commonly used ambulatory aids. A: Cane. B: Quad cane. C: Forearm crutch.

D

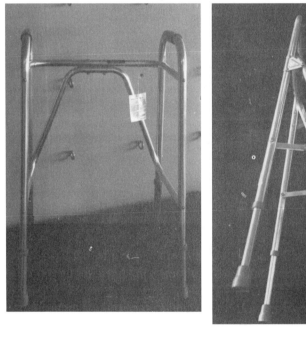

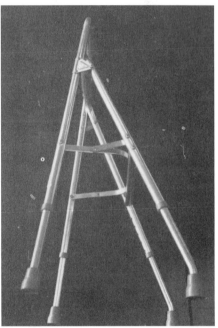

E   **F**

FIGURE 2.8 (CONTINUED). Commonly used ambulatory aids. **D:** Ankle-foot orthoses (AFO). **E:** Walker. **F:** Walkane.

Bracing

The most common braces used to brace the lower extremities in MS are standard polypropylene AFOs and those with an articulated joint. The following guidelines may be helpful.

A standard AFO (Fig. 2.8) is indicated if the patient exhibits
1. Consistent foot drop or toe drag
2. Poor knee control (especially hyperextension)
3. Weakness of grade 2 or 3 at the ankle with dorsiflexion testing
4. Minimal-to-moderate spasticity
5. Poor endurance in gait
6. Poor proprioception and sensory sense

The advantages of an AFO are that it
1. Saves energy during gait because the patient does not work as hard to clear his/her toes during the swing through phase of the gait
2. Improves foot drop or toe drag during the swing phase of gait
3. Improves general safety during walking by avoiding many falls due to the toe drag
4. Provides more knee control during mid-stance phase of gait by avoiding hyperextension of the knee
5. Provides greater ankle stability
6. Improves the overall gait pattern
7. Provides better cosmesis for the patient

The advantages of the AFO with an articulating joint are
1. All of the above listed for the standard AFO.
2. It allows some mobility at the ankle joint. This permits a more natural movement at the ankle during gait, which looks more normal. It allows the patient to drive while wearing the brace, and allows more freedom for squatting down in order to reach objects on the floor.
3. It provides a plantar flexion stop to prevent the foot from further plantar flexion during swing phase of gait.
4. It still allows for dorsiflexion assist, and can be set up to 5 degrees of dorsiflexion to clear the foot during the swing through phase.

Relative contraindications for these types of braces are
1. Moderate or severe spasticity in the lower extremities
2. Severe foot edema
3. Severe weakness (muscles grades 2 or less) at the hips

A double upright metal brace can provide some of the same advantages listed above, and usually provides more adjustments for the ankle and the knee. However, this brace is usually not the preferred choice due to its weight and poorer cosmetic appearance.

The polypropylene AFOs may be set in a few degrees of dorsiflexion to provide better knee control. If hyperextension is severe, a Swedish hyperextension knee cage may be useful. In some people this device may be quite helpful, but it is decidedly more bulky and often moves down the leg, which decreases its effectiveness. Custom bracing of the knee can be the answer to this problem, as effective orthotics may make up for instability of the joints, tendons, and ligaments. This usually requires the skills of a trained orthotist and is a topic beyond the scope of this book.

Some therapists have found rocker clog shoes to be of some help for those few people who need to have the plantar flexed position neutralized while the curved forefoot sole will initiate knee flexion. A skilled therapist should determine if this situation is present before purchase of this device is recommended.

WHEELCHAIRS

Wheelchair prescribing is both an art and a science. There are no absolute rules unique to MS. For a detailed discussion of this topic, refer to Wheelchairs: A Prescription Guide, by A. Bennett Wilson (1990). Discussed below are some general guidelines regarding types of wheelchairs and seating.

While the patient is seated in a wheelchair observe the following characteristics:

1. Is the head held up at the midline?
2. Are the shoulders at equal height?
3. Is the patient hunched forward?
4. Is the patient leaning to one side?

5. Is one hip higher than the other?
6. Are the knees raised or sloping toward the floor?
7. Are the footrests at the same height?
8. Is the patient in a "slumped" or "sliding out" position?

A patient may be sitting in misalignment due to degenerative changes, contractures, muscle weakness, or to an incorrectly adjusted wheelchair. The basics of positioning start with moving the pelvis and spinal column/head into correct alignment, then aligning the limbs. The pelvis should be in a neutral alignment in all three axes of space. It should not be tilted forward or backward, to the right or left, and should not be twisted in either direction around the spinal column. The spinal column should be upright and the head centered. A normal spinal column has a slight outward curve at the cervical spine and a slight inward curve at the lumbar spine.

The wheelchair seating system can be modified by adding commercially available components or by switching to a contoured seating system that is customized to the individual (Fig. 2.9). Adding components such as plywood or foam inserts, or clamp-on side supports, usually works well for MS patients, who do not generally have severe musculoskeletal deformities. Customized, contoured seating systems use specific materials and techniques to mold the seat around the patient, while s/he is held in correct body alignment. This process take 2–4 hours and produces a template that is shipped to the manufacturer to make a more substantial model. The patient is later evaluated in that model to see if further modifications are necessary. These systems are expensive, and therapists must be trained in their use.

A standard wheelchair is appropriate for the patient who has sufficient strength to hold his/her head and body erect. A cushion should always be used to relieve ischial and sacral pressure. If weakness increases, a different cushion should be chosen to maintain the pelvis in a correct position, clamp-on thoracic supports can be added to maintain an erect spinal column, a head/neck rest can be attached to support the head at the midline, and calf supports or heel loops can be used to keep the foot on the footrest. The footrest height should be adjusted so that the thighs are parallel with the floor.

If the patient tends to slide out of the chair, a cushion with a molded depression for the buttocks, or a 10-degree wedge under his/her present cushion, may relieve the problem. However, these may put increased pressure on the sacral area. A seat belt placed across the thighs (rather than across the pelvis) may be helpful. A semireclining wheelchair is also appropriate for a patient who appears to be "slumped" or is sliding out of the chair. If the patient tends to lean to one side due to weakness, foam inserts or clamp-on thoracic supports can be used to keep the spinal column in alignment. If the patient sits "hunched forward," with the shoulders protracted and head down, a standard wheelchair with head/neck support and a soft foam cervical collar may work. A semireclining wheelchair is often most effective in bringing the head into line with the spinal column.

There are no hard and fast rules to choosing a cushion, and a patient's cushioning needs may change with time. Because the prevention of skin breakdown is of overwhelming medical importance, cushions that provide adequate pressure relief should be considered first.

Patients may be categorized into low-, medium-, or high-risk groups for developing skin breakdown. Those who are able to do a standing transfer and can shift their weight easily and naturally when seated are at low risk. Patients who cannot do a standing transfer, but who conscientiously do pressure relief exercises and are properly

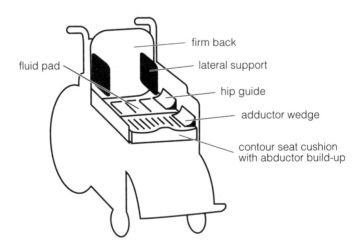

FIGURE 2.9. Some wheelchair adaptations.

nourished, are in the medium-risk group. In the high-risk group are patients who need assistance to perform pressure relief exercises and who may sit for long periods of time without relieving pressure.

Cushions for patients in the low and medium risk groups include those made of dense foam, such as T-Foam®, or foam and gel combination such as Akros® or Aquatherm® cushions. A solid seat and/or solid back insert can be used to overcome the sling effect of vinyl wheelchair upholstery.

A gel cushion such as the Jay®, or a foam cut-out cushion such as the Postureform® or Laminaire®, are appropriate for patients in the medium- and high-risk groups. For some patients a RoHo® air cushion has worked well, but these require more care as punctures must be avoided and proper inflation maintained. Again, a solid seat/back insert should be considered with all but the Jay® cushion.

The Jay® cushion has a semisolid base to which an envelope of gel is attached with Velcro. A polyester cover fits over the base and the gel. A special "quadrant filled" gel envelope restricts movement of the gel and is recommended for use with reclining wheelchairs. Jay Medical also makes a wedge that can be inserted under any cushion.

Laminaire® and Posturform® cushions consist of two layers of foam glued together. The Postureform® cushion has a rear cut-out to relieve pressure in the ischial and sacral areas. The Laminaire® cushion is customized to each patient; the therapist makes the foam cut-out (an electric knife is recommended to cut the foam) guided by readings from a pressure evaluator made by the Scimedics® Corporation; this evaluator is a small plastic disc that is placed between the seated patient and the cushion. The patient's wheelchair should be adjusted with footrests at the correct height, and an incontinence protection cover should be in place over the cushion if needed. The evaluator indicates the amount of pressure, in millimeters of mercury, that the body is exerting against the cushion. As the therapist makes repeatedly deeper cut-outs in the foam, the pressure reading falls into the desired range, usually about 40 mm/Hg under the ischial tuberosities. The pressure evaluator can be used to measure the amount of pressure the seated patient exerts against any cushion, thus measuring its effectiveness in preventing skin breakdown.

Simple air and water cushions should be avoided because they are easily punctured. Furthermore, water as a supporting medium produces a shearing effect between layers of skin tissue. Any cushion's effectiveness should be regularly re-evaluated every 3-6 months, or if the patient reports a reddened or darkened skin area.

The likelihood of a patient developing skin breakdown can be greatly reduced by good general nutrition, correct positioning, an appropriate cushion, and pressure relief exercises done for a few minutes two or three times an hour.

PHYSICAL FITNESS

The term physical fitness refers to enhanced physiological or functional capacity, which allows for an improved quality of life. It is important to everyone, whether or not they have MS. The capacity for exercise increases with increasing physical or functional capacity, as reflected by physiological adaptations that include a lowered heart rate and improved mobility during exercise. A good quality of life involves an overall positive feeling and enthusiasm for life, without the development of fatigue or exhaustion from routine activity.

Human performance is the result of many components of sensory and motor interaction, mediated by cognitive and other central processes. Sedentary individuals have a reduced capacity and tolerance for exercise. Activity limitation, regardless of its cause, results in a functional decline of the cardiovascular and pulmonary systems. Conversely, physical activity is required to maintain the body's cardiovascular and pulmonary systems at optimal levels of function.

Activity restriction results in a general deconditioning, a decline in physical fitness that is referred to as a hypokinetic disorder. This is directly attributed to motion deficiency, and produces the following symptoms: (1) increased neuromuscular tension, (2) increased pulse rate at rest, (3) decreased adrenocortical reserve, (4) decreased muscular strength, (5) decreased vital capacity at rest, (6) decreased maximum vital capacity, (7) increased fatigue, (8) increased anxiety, and (9) increased depression.

The benefits of aerobic exercise are related to the increased utilization of oxygen to generate chemical energy. Cells use energy from food by breaking down the chemical compound known as adenosine triphosphate (ATP). ATP is the immediate usable form of chemical energy needed for cellular function including muscular contraction. Some ATP is used immediately following food breakdown, while some is stored in cells for future use. ATP may be produced aerobically or anaerobically. However, the aerobic production of ATP is slower because it requires continuous oxygen to the metabolically active cells. The byproducts of aerobic metabolism, carbon dioxide and water, do not cause fatigue. Thus, this pathway is limited only by substrate (glucose stored as glycogen and fat) depletion. Depletion will not occur until two or more continuous hours of exercise are completed. The aerobic production of ATP is more efficient than the anaerobic, and yields a considerably higher amount of ATP per unit of substrate.

A positive factor in anaerobic ATP production is that it does not require the presence of oxygen; thus it can be used immediately. However, there are many negative factors, which are especially a problem in the MS population. Very little energy is produced relative to the amount of substrate utilized. Also, because only glucose can be used as a substrate, substrate depletion is a limiting factor. In addition, the byproduct of anaerobic metabolism is lactic acid, which induces fatigue when present in the muscle tissue .

The energy for most types of exercise comes from a combination of aerobic and anaerobic sources. Initially, exercise relies more heavily on anaerobic metabolism. Once a steady state occurs, the body switches to a dependence on aerobic metabolism. However, the exercise turns anaerobic again if its intensity becomes too high.

Aerobic exercise typically should be low to moderate in intensity and involve the large muscle groups moving continuously, without producing undue respiratory distress. An exercise program should be tailored to each individual, rather than simply prescribing a general program which will fail to fit the individual. A low-to-moderate intensity of aerobic exercise is recommended for MS patients. The "no pain, no gain" approach will result in failure.

The benefits of aerobic exercise can be divided according to what occurs physiologically. Aerobic exercise, carried out appropriately, improves the musculoskeletal system by

- Increasing lean muscle mass
- Increasing flexibility

- Increasing muscle tone
- Decreasing body fat content

Cardiac improvements include
- Decreased heart rate at rest and with exercise
- Increased heart rate recovery following exercise
- Increased stroke volume (blood volume with each beat of the heart)
- Increased cardiac contraction
- Increased heart size
- Increased blood supply to the heart tissue.

Improvements in respiratory function include
- Increased functional capacity (maximum inspiration to maximum expiration)
- Increased tidal volume (volume of air either during inspiration or expiration)
- Increased respiratory ventilation

Aerobic exercise can also result in
- Beneficial changes to blood vessels and blood chemistry
- Decreases in resting blood pressures
- Decreases in serum levels of lipids or fats accompanied by increases in blood volume and the blood supply to the muscles

Finally, psychological benefits derived from aerobic exercise include increases in vigor, self esteem, concentration, academic performance, and sleep quality, and decreases in anxiety and depression.

Until recently, suggesting exercise for the treatment of MS would have initiated a rash of criticism from medical professionals, who felt that the problems of fatigue and poor endurance in MS patients were insurmountable obstacles to exercise training. Medical concerns that an increase in symptoms or a potential relapse might occur justified the advice to "take it easy and avoid exertion." However, it is now understood that appropriate exercise training may result in improved self-image and function, and that the effects of inactivity may amplify disease morbidity. Fear and over-reaction may lead to increased disability, causing the patient to function below capacity. This sequence of events is the result of increased autonomic activity with an outpouring of adrenalin and the increased potential for "clutching" under the stress.

It is common for patients to harbor expectations of normal activity long after the development of MS symptoms and its diagnosis. They may feel driven to attempt activities beyond their true ability, resulting in magnification of their symptoms. An appropriately prescribed program of exercise training provides the patient with the necessary tools to monitor his/her physical status and to make necessary accurate adjustments in daily activities and self imposed limitations.

Taking control of one's health may be the most important focus of the person with MS. Success in this area may partially offset the frustrations and limitations of living with a chronic progressive disease, and provide an uplifting outlook that can in turn, improve the patient's quality of life.

Exercise

EXERCISE PRESCRIPTION

All exercise recommendations must be based on a detailed medical and physical evaluation. This evaluation has two primary objectives: to identify the patient's current physical and medical status as related to the presence of MS and the ability to perform exercise, and to serve as an objective baseline for developing an exercise prescription to begin training and make future reference to document status change. The prescription provides the technical, medical, and physiological basis for an exercise training program that will maximize the patient's health, and should recommend the safest and most effective strategies to achieve individual goals. A detailed exercise prescription represents the summation of all the medical and clinical data collected and sets forth the training guidelines for that individual. The prescription should be modified frequently to accommodate changes in physical and medical status. It includes: (1) a goals statement, (2) a statement of purpose and objectives of exercise, (3) recommendations of specific types of exercise, and (4) principles of training, including intensity, frequency, duration, progression, apparatus, assistance, and recuperation.

Good examples of aerobic exercise that utilize the large muscle groups in a continuous fashion include walking, jogging, biking, rowing, swimming pool exercises, cross-country skiing, and low impact aerobic dance exercise.

Endurance limitations in MS include fatigue, leg discomfort, dizziness, weakness, confusion, exercise test duration, physical work capacity, pulmonary function, respiration, autonomic function (heart rate response, blood pressure response), and motor control.

To be aerobic, walking and/or jogging and cross-country skiing require adequate balance, coordination, and strength for movement at recommended speeds. Stationary exercise equipment such as bikes and rowing machines provide an exercise option for individuals with balance and coordination problems. Stationary bicycles that utilize contralateral upper extremity and lower extremity action are excellent choices of equipment. They allow for total body exercise, which is advantageous for those with paresis or paralysis in any of the extremities.

EXERCISE TESTING

For the general public, exercise testing should follow accepted principles as adopted by the American College of Sports Medicine. The recommended exercise intensity is 50 to 80 percent of the maximum adjusted heart rate. Target heart rate zones are a fairly reliable indicator of training intensity and commonly used rather than measurement of maximum oxygen uptake (aerobic capacity) which is costly and time consuming. Exercise below the target zone range results in little if any training, while exercise above this range becomes anaerobic.

MS patients almost never test to the maximum oxygen uptake due to MS fatigue and related problems associated with maximum exercise. An understanding of this is key to developing exercise programs for these patients.

Exercise target heart rate guidelines are used in conjunction with several other measurements. Breathing is continuously assessed for the onset of hyperventilation, clinically determined by the inability to say a phrase of three to five words without requiring a breath. This is approximately the point at which aerobic exercise becomes anaerobic and the exercise evaluation should be terminated. The sensation of hyperventilation should be pointed out to the MS patient to increase its familiarity and recognition of the symptoms in future sessions.

Another tool utilized to assess exercise tolerance is the Borg Scale of Perceived Exertion, in which numeric values are assigned to the degree of fatigue. Individuals are asked to rate the exercise intensity according to this scale. Following completion of the exercise evaluation, heart rates and Perceived Exertion Ratings correlating to the stage prior to hyperventilation should be appropriate for aerobic conditioning intensity.

Another important characteristic of aerobic exercise is its duration, which is optimally thirty minutes. However, it is advisable to begin with a shorter duration that is within the patient's own tolerance level and to then build up gradually. Individuals whose condition is poor can derive benefits from even 5–10 minutes of exercise. MS persons must be cautioned to modify exercise intensities and duration if illness or exacerbations of the disease occur.

The frequency of exercise sessions is important. Generally, three to four times per week is considered optimal while two to three times per week is a minimum. Frequency is not as important as duration or intensity. Research has not shown any statistically significant difference between two versus four times per week or three versus five times per week. With increases in frequency the individual will have a higher risk of developing musculoskeletal injury. It is important to determine one's goals and to increase gradually.

All aerobic exercise sessions must begin with a warm-up and be completed with a cool-down. The patient must understand that these should never be omitted. The warm-up increases circulation, augmenting oxygen delivery to the muscles and increasing body temperature, which in turn increases the efficiency of muscle contraction. A warm-up optimizes attainment of "second wind" by assisting in the response of the circulation, respiratory, and musculoskeletal systems, and also reduces ischemia. The increased flexibility resulting from stretching decreases the possibility of musculoskeletal injury and alleviates muscle soreness. While a warm-up period is essential, it is also important to understand that a rise in core body temperature results in inefficient nerve conduction and weakness. *This over-heating must be avoided.*

A properly performed cool-down decreases the risk of musculoskeletal injury and myocardial ischemia/arrhythmias, and reduces muscle soreness. The cardiovascular cool-down replenishes energy reserves and transports waste byproducts such as lactic acid out of the muscle tissues. The cool-down also assists in preventing venous pooling in the lower extremities, which may result in hypotension.

Patients with MS should return for followup visits and review the exercise prescription with the therapist. The exercise diary, an exercise log of the patient's individual exercise program, should be reviewed for exercise modalities of choice, intensity, duration, and frequency. Methods of pulse monitoring and the patient's understanding of the Borg Scale of Perceived Exertion are also reviewed. Suggestions and motivation are given to ensure continued consistency, and ultimately success, with a lifetime of aerobic exercise.

SUMMARY The MS patient must be prepared to train if an exercise program is to be effective. Preparation considers the following areas:

ATTITUDE: A positive commitment to improving health is a prerequisite for successful exercise training; the MS patient must accept an improved health status as his/her personal challenge and actively pursue exercise as a means to that goal.

EVALUATION: The MS patient should be instructed in the techniques of self-evaluation to monitor daily fluctuations in functional and neurological status.

EDUCATION: The MS patient must understand exercise and its relation to health endeavors; s/he must be informed and capable of establishing realistic objectives regarding health expectations; knowing how to exercise, when to exercise, and the proper clothing to wear should be reinforced and stressed repeatedly by the therapist.

EXERCISE PRESCRIPTION: The prescription must be clear, concise, and explicitly in establishing guidelines for training; it should be accomplished with reasonable effort and build upon successes.

CONVENIENCE: Daily routines and activities should be arranged to make exercise convenient and yet afford ample time for work and leisure pursuits.

HABIT: Exercise should become habitual; a psychological dependency on exercising should be viewed as favorable.

Recreation

MS patients can also pursue various recreational activities if the following is kept in mind:

1. Plan for the temperature and time of day.
2. Develop awareness of physical responses that indicate maximum tolerable activity has been reached.
3. Slowly increase endurance for a specific activity.
4. Learn to monitor fatigue level.

The therapist can provide helpful information to adapt some of these activities to a specific MS patient's needs. Recreational activities that have been successful include yoga, pool therapy, and adapted skiing. Supervision by a therapist in many of these activities ensures safety and emphasizes the therapeutic effects of these programs in MS. Patients with minimal or moderate disabilities seem to receive the greatest physical benefit from these activities, although some with severe disabilities may find them helpful as well.

AQUATIC EXERCISE

Because of the natural buoyancy of water, an aquatic program allows patients to exercise more easily, walk with less difficulty, relax spastic muscles, and practice balance activities more safely. A swimming program can also contribute to improving strength and endurance. The following therapeutic exercise programs can be performed easily in the water:

- Specific strengthening protocols for the upper extremities, trunk, and lower extremities
- Stretching exercises to increase flexibility
- Swimming endurance programs for general conditioning as well as decreasing fatigue
- Simple ambulatory skills to improve gait and endurance
- Complex movement pattern performance for improving coordination and balance.

In all these programs, water can be used to provide assistance, resistance, and support. Aquatic exercise provides full range of motion resistance at varying speeds to enhance the strengthening of specific muscle groups. The turbulence of the water enhances central stabilization by providing co-contraction of the abdominals and back muscles, and may result in improved trunk control. Of great importance in MS, the effects of exercising in cool water minimizes the effects of heat from exercising, a major problem for some MS patients. In addition, the cool temperature of the water (80-85 degrees Fahrenheit) will generally first decrease heart rate and then increase it in proportion to the intensity of the exercise. Consequently, a greater level of exercise can be tolerated in the water, while maintaining a lower heart rate and thus achieving higher levels of aerobic conditioning. There are also social and psychological benefits to an aquatic program. The comraderie developed among patients provides for long-lasting relationships and can serve as their support group. Experiencing success with an aquatic program may help a patient to have a positive attitude about other areas in life, and the success and enjoyment of this type of exercise can contribute to compliance with a long term exercise program.

YOGA

Yoga programs for MS patients can help improve flexibility, strength, and coordination, and also teach valuable relaxation techniques. Some yoga postures may have to be adapted to specific patients' needs. Having a therapist available during a yoga class is extremely valuable in adapting exercises and in monitoring spasticity, fatigue, weakness, or balance problems for each participant.

SKIING

An adapted ski program offers some of the same benefits as yoga, and offers a positive and enjoyable outdoor experience as well. With adaptive equipment and special instruction, the patient has the opportunity to enjoy a sport usually perceived as being only for the physically fit. Patients can develop better balance and increased endurance as well as the confidence to try other activities in their own life. Fatigue can be an important factor with all these activities; the patient needs to be aware of this and learn to manage it effectively.

MUSCULOSKELETAL DYSFUNCTION

MS may affect the musculoskeletal system indirectly, producing complications that are as varied as the direct symptoms of MS. These complications may cause great discomfort and should be managed aggressively.

Hammer toes, foot inversion, and increased plantar flexion may occur secondary to spasticity, resulting in significant gait abnormalities.

Decreased control accompanied by decreased sensation in the legs may result in overuse syndromes. These include a variety of musculoskeletal problems associated with the knee. Chronic hyperextension from imbalance of muscle strength or incoordination may damage the posterior ligaments of the knee. The resulting knee pain and weakness may further affect an already unstable gait pattern. A knee brace will help prevent damage to the posterior ligaments of the knee due to chronic hyperextension.

As a detailed discussion of these complications is beyond the scope of this book, the reader is referred to the major textbooks of neurology, rehabilitation, and orthopedics for more extensive discussion of their management.

The normal functioning of the hip and sacral area also depend on a balance of the surrounding muscles. An imbalance due to MS may result in sacral torsion or annominate rotation; pain in the hip area then results in an inefficient walking pattern.

The most common musculoskeletal complaint in MS is chronic low back pain. Often the patient's posture is poor, producing a loss of lumbar lordosis. Fatigue exacerbates this problem. Poor balance can create a forward flexion at the hips and add to the development of chronic back pain. Paraspinal spasticity can also cause chronic low back pain.

At times it is difficult, even for the trained neurologist, to distinguish radicular appearing pain from demylination adjacent to the dorsal root ganglia, giving the appearance of a herniated disc. A burning quality of the radiating pain may indicate MS whereas a decreased reflex may indicate mechanical, discogenic disease. When in question, further diagnostic tests are necessary, which may include neurologic evaluation, electromyography, magnetic resonance imaging, or computerized tomography.

The therapist must be alert to the fact that there may be additional treatable rehabilitative problems in the MS patient that may or may not be related to MS. These must be identified and managed to allow for productive rehabilitation.

3

OCCUPATIONAL THERAPY

CHARLOTTE BHASIN, M.O.T., O.T.R./L., DONNA JENSEN, O.T.R., MARY LENLING, O.T.R., KATE ROBBINS, O.T.R., AND RANDALL T. SCHAPIRO, M.D.

The orchestration of willful, directed, skilled, fine motor activity is dependent on the integrity of the nervous system at all levels. Disruption by multiple sclerosis (MS) scars (plaques) will alter the timing, intensity, direction, and location of sensory motor signals, wreaking havoc on this precise system.

EVALUATION

Definition

Occupational therapists are concerned with how one is "occupied" in daily life. When disease disrupts the usual routine, occupational therapy can be instrumental in assessing and developing alternative methods to continue with the routines of daily life. Because so much skilled activity is carried out with the hands and arms, occupational therapists have become specialized in treating hand and arm dysfunction. Despite this, it is truly a misnomer to label occupational therapists as only "arm" therapists. As all therapists, occupational therapists are interested in the whole person and in functional improvement at all anatomic levels.

Evaluation of the upper extremities documents baseline performance for future comparison and identifies areas that are potentially remediable or for which compensatory techniques can be used. This evaluation should be done upon admission or re-admission as either an outpatient or inpatient, since records of past performance provide valuable data on which treatment protocols may be based.

The assessment should include the date of diagnosis, reason for testing, current living situation, responsibilities in the home, family structure, vocation, avocational interests, cognition history, wheelchair positioning needs, and both subjective and objective assessments of activities of daily living (ADL).

Evaluation of Sensory Systems

Numbness, pain, and other sensory aberrations frequently are present in the upper extremities of people with MS. This directly influences the quality of information transmitted between the sensory-motor pathways and the brain. Since discriminitive sensations are required for most fine motor tasks, the focus of the initial evaluation should be in this area. Functionally, discrimination may be tested by stereognostic evaluation. Unfortunately, there are no normative data or accepted standardized procedures for this type of testing. The Occupational Therapy Section of the Mellen Center for MS at the Cleveland Clinic Foundation has developed the following standardized procedures and rating scale:

A lid with a sampling of small objects is left in full view of the patient, and a duplicate set of objects is used by the therapist. The patient is told: "I'm going to hide one of your hands behind this folder and then give you one of those objects from my box. Without looking, I want you to feel the object and tell me which one you think is in your hand." The sample objects are left in full view throughout the test to eliminate the word finding/naming difficulties that can result from cognitive changes and skew the test results. The patient answers and the examiner responds with, "Good." to each response, correct or incorrect. Results are shared with the patients only after testing the second hand to reduce guessing.

Minor cognitive changes are often apparent during this testing, including mislabeling and paraphasic errors. As long as the patient points to the correct object, the response is counted as correct. If the patient both misnames and mispoints, the response is incorrect.

The right hand is consecutively presented with a paperclip, dime, and quarter; the left hand with a nickel, medium safety pin, and penny. These objects were chosen to reflect shape discrimination between the coins and wire objects, as well as size discrimination and edge roughness.

Scoring is as follows:

Intact: All correct, with response given within 10 seconds of object presentation.
Impaired: One wrong or two wrong or longer than 10 seconds on two out of three responses, even if correct.
Absent: None correct.

The same objects are always presented in the same order to the same hand on all subsequent retests. In the absence of definitive norms, this allows for objective comparison between two points in time for the same person.

Another quantifiable sensory test is two-point discrimination, which uses an aestheiometer, caliper, or hemming ruler. The patient must be reliable in terms of providing accurate responses for meaningful data to be obtained. The methods for two-point discrimination involve the simultaneous application to the skin of two blunted or rounded points, applied at decreasing distances apart until the two stimuli are perceived as one. The patient is not to look as the testing is done. Norms vary, but 2–6 mm is generally accepted as the normal range. When the two points cannot be discriminated at or below 7 mm, patients complain of dropping light objects without being aware of their dropping; by 8–9 mm, there are complaints of significant hand numbness; and at 10 mm, dense hand numbness that interferes with hand function is described. Subjectively, the quality of the movements and their effects on writing, feeding, dressing, etc., should be documented.

Evaluation of Upper Extremity Strength and Motion

Strength is defined as the "brute force" of an isolated muscle group, independent of the quality of movement made by the muscle group; this distinguishes strength from coordination. The two factors in MS that contribute to weakness in the upper extremity are decreased nerve transmission due to an upper motor neuron lesion and muscle atrophy secondary to disuse.

The Manual Muscle Test (MMT) is widely used for evaluating strength, although it has a low inter-relater reliability. It is, however, a viable method for gross distinction of strength when performed by the same examiner over time. The precursor to testing individual muscles is to determine active and passive range of motion, so that range limitations are known before force is applied. It is important to note that a score of 5/5, or "good," obtained in MMT is not always a "normal" muscle, because the MMT tests only one maximal contraction; it does not detect fatigue, which occurs with repeated contractions as seen in MS.

Hand-strength testing should be done in a standardized manner, as norms are only meaningful if the procedures are followed exactly. Standardized arm position, the sequence of testing positions (with the dynamometer reading the last whole line to the left of the red max hand needle), and the taking the average (mean) of three trials are essential for proper interpretation.

Quantification of the raw score is important. The calculation of z-scores can be useful clinically, particularly in tracking status across time. The z-score represents the number of standard deviations a raw score is from the known mean of the population sample. It represents distance from the "average" score for a person of the same sex, using the same hand, with no physical abnormality. An MS patient's score may continue to be "abnormal," but knowing that strength went from a z-score of -2.0 to -4.0 will allow for inferences regarding the degree of weakness. With the use of only raw scores, for example, a hand-strength measurement showing a drop of 53 to 43 pounds cannot allow for interpretation of significance. Misinterpretation leads to inaccurate treatment focus.

Hand dominance should also be determined, since many MS patients have been forced to change hands due to tremor or weakness, or to use both hands for different activities. Therefore, grip strength (dynameter) and pinch strength (pinch meter) should also be tested. These results can be compared against norms, compared right against left, and compared against earlier evaluations. The presence of spasticity can significantly affect the results; for scoring and discussion of spasticity (see Spasticity in Chapter 2).

It is important to emphasize that problems of range of motion and muscle tone can influence strength testing. Strength measurements must therefore be qualified by statements about abnormalities of range of motion (ROM) and muscle tone.

TREATMENT OF UPPER EXTREMITY WEAKNESS

Treatment of upper extremity weakness should be done slowly, in a graded manner, always with the understanding that progressive resistive exercises will result in fatigue and increased weakness, not strength, in a muscle weakened by the denervation of central demyelination. Therapeutic activities for the weakened upper extremity should be designed to reinforce the use of the muscles to be strengthened or to develop compensatory motor patterns to replace function lost through weakness. Principles of grading activity through positioning (horizontal vs. inclined vs. vertical planes, and distance from the patient), no resistance to maximal resistance, gross to fine motor, and knowledge of muscles or muscle groups utilized should be incorporated into the treatment design and selection of exercises and activities. When attempting to substitute for lost muscle strength, the therapist should attempt to locate and to "harness" any available muscles, and utilize external devices to replace lost function. For example, in the absence of spasticity, an overhead suspension sling or mobile arm support may be used to substitute for weak shoulder and elbow flexors. Results will be better when tremor and trunk weakness do not interfere. Initially, any exercise should be lightly resistive to observe its effect, using therabands (not indicated with increased tone), wrist weights, or theraplast for the hand. Progression should only be as rapid as can be tolerated. Getting the "disused muscle" back into use is important and may take innovation. Fatigue should be avoided:

increasing repetitions rather than increasing weight is recommended. The exercise program should be taught in conjunction with functional use of the affected muscle and with energy conservation tips for upper extremity activities, i.e., rest breaks when writing, eliminating high reaching into cupboards, the use of adaptive devices.

If pronounced weakness in the hands and arms limits the active range of motion, passive range of motion should be utilized to maintain joint mobility and to reduce the possibility of capsule adhesions. Responsibility for ROM exercise should be turned over to the patient when possible by training in self-ROM. If the patient is unable to carry out the exercise program, a caregiver should be trained to do the ROM.

Static splinting may be used to maintain proper hand positioning if the finger and wrist extensors are weak. Unless strong flexor tone is present, resting splints should be worn only at night. Their use should not be a substitution for passive range of motion; both are needed to maintain hand positioning and joint and tendon elasticity. In the presence of increased tone, air splints worn during or outside of treatments for a maximum of 30 minutes can be of assistance in reducing or controlling abnormal tone. They are available in a range of lengths from wrist/ankle to full arm or full leg, to encompass more than one joint. For the upper extremity, apply the splint after positioning the limb in external rotation, elbow and wrist extension, finger extension, and thumb abduction. Small adjustments are easily made to reposition any joint, by reducing the air pressure, repositioning, then increasing the inflation of the splint. Of particular benefit is the inclusion of the extended elbow in the splint during weightbearing involving the upper extremity. Patients and family readily learn application and removal and frequency of use. This can be incorporated into an overall home program of muscle tone control.

Coordination

Coordination involves the timing of movements in multiple muscle groups to produce a skilled, voluntary movement. This involves multiple muscle movements, and no single assessment procedure will test them all. In the interest of efficiency, decisions must be made when testing the person with MS.

Because fine motor control of the hand represents the highest level of coordinated sensory-motor integration in the upper extremity, its evaluation begins the decision-making process for further evaluation. The Nine-Hole Peg Test (Mathiowetz et al., 1985) is used to screen for coordination. Performance on this quick test allows for the determination of whether further in-depth coordination testing with a variety of parameters is necessary.

The test must be administered properly to be reliable and valid. Sources of error arise when, in the interest of time, only one trial per hand is given rather than two. The faster of the two trials is the actual raw score, not the average of the two. z-scores should be calculated to determine the distance from the population mean, as was done with hand strength testing; a 20% or greater change in a patient's raw score is indicative of a true change in function (Goodkin, 1988). The Box and Blocks Test (Mathiowetz et al., 1985) gives another objective measurement which can be followed over time to determine both gross dexterity and upper extremity endurance.

After the fine motor standardized screening testing, the initial evaluation must consider the overall quality of movement of the upper extremity. Movement patterns of the patient when performing fine motor functional tasks such as threading a needle, using scissors, handling utensils, buttoning, or using small hand tools must be observed and documented.

Spasticity adds to the problems produced by an intention tremor and leads to increased problems in measuring ataxia. Thus, if at all possible, the effects of spasticity should be minimized through such methods as positioning techniques. In addition, since visual dysfunction is common in MS and has a definite impact on hand coordination, tests of coordination should be preceded by a gross visual function test.

Once the initial evaluation has screened both fine and gross motor quality of movement, later testing can be used to serve as a baseline for setting treatment goals. Some tests that have been helpful include the Jebsen Test of Hand Function, Minnesota Rate of Manipulation (MRMT), The Purdue Pegboard, and typing speed and accuracy.

In summary, the spectrum of upper extremity dysfunction includes input from sensation, vision, strength, and coordination, all of which need to be tested. All tests, and the conclusions drawn from them must take into consideration the interrelationships that make the arms and hands function appropriately.

Treatment of Upper Extremity Incoordination and Tremor

When evaluating tremors it is therapeutically important to determine whether they are proximal, distal, or both. Stabilization for tremor control can be done in a variety of ways. Air splints can be worn to stabilize the elbow and/or arm and keep the hand free to write or paint. Weighted eating utensils and cups are sometimes helpful in decreasing tremors during eating. Sometimes a change of hand dominance is necessary if one upper extremity is more tremulous than the other. Splints can be fabricated to stabilize the wrists, keeping the fingers free. A soft cervical collar may help stabilize the head. Lateral supports in a wheelchair help stabilize the trunk, allowing the upper extremities to have freer movement. Experimentation with one or many of these ideas is usually needed before any degree of success is achieved.

FATIGUE

Fatigue is one of the most common symptoms in MS, but it is paid far too little attention because it is invisible to a casual observer. This leads to frustration for the patient, as others often conclude that s/he is either seeking attention or being lazy.

Fatigue may in fact be the most disabling symptom experienced by the person with MS, and everyone involved in its treatment must be aware of the problems that fatigue can create, including both poor physical prowess and as increased cognitive difficulties. The neurologist may recommend medication; the dietitian and speech pathologist may suggest that the patient eat foods with a specific constituency to decrease fatigue produced by eating; the physical therapist may try to build endurance or increase the efficiency of walking and other activities; and the occupational therapist often will take special interest in how individuals plan the day and function with the activities of daily living. Dealing with fatigue may be as simple as suggesting that the patient do more in the morning when energy level is higher, or it may involve detailed testing and individualized planning.

It is important to understand and differentiate the types of fatigue found in MS in order to treat it appropriately.

Normal Fatigue: This type of fatigue is experienced by everyone after rigorous activity. It is managed simply by understanding its cause and making appropriate adjustments in behavior.

"Short Circuiting" Fatigue: This is seen in some individuals who have demyelinated nerves, which fatigue with use. These individuals may start walking normally but their leg(s) fail to function after a short distance. This type of fatigue must be managed by appropriate rest periods that allow nerve function to be restored.

Depression: Depression leads to sleep disturbances, appetite disturbances and fatigue. It is treated with antidepressants and counselling.

Lassitude: This term is applied to those with "MS fatigue," which involves a feeling of sleepiness after almost no activity. This type of fatigue comes on suddenly and is often overpowering. Individuals with this type of fatigue will sometimes respond to amantidine (Symmetrel), pemoline (Cylert), or other pharmacologic management.

In dealing with any type of fatigue, it is helpful to apply energy conservation techniques, time management principles, and to perform activities in the most efficient manner.

CONCEPT OF TIME

In order to conserve energy, efficiency is a necessity in MS. Thus, an understanding of time management is essential to effective planning. Reviewing a few facts about time will make this process clearer:

1. There is no such thing as lack of time—there are 24 hours in each day.

2. No one other than the individual controls his/her time.
3. Each individual has a different perspective on time, which is influenced by personality, education, and culture.
4. It is the responsibility of each individual to choose how to use time.
5. Understanding that control over time gives control over life can reduce stress.

Myths About Time

The efficient use of time is particularly important to the person with MS. There are many myths about time that are easily accepted, and which hinder ones' efforts to use time efficiently. Some of the most common myths about time are dispelled below.

1. *Those who are the most active get the most done.* This myth confuses activity with results: running around in a flurry usually accomplishes little.
2. *If I do it myself it will be done faster and better than if anyone else does it.* This is a myth because it results in the individual doing everything: teaching others how to do certain tasks lessens the burden on one individual.
3. *The harder one works, the more work accomplished.* This is a myth because hard work alone does not ensure that things will get done: being well organized in working toward a goal is more effective.
4. *Time can be "saved."* Time can never be saved—only better utilized through planning and organization.
5. *Time is against us.* Time cannot "fight"—people fight by mismanaging time.

Control over time does not necessarily lead to success. It does mean responsibility and should be taught in that light. Having a sense of control over life does not necessarily lead to enjoyment, but it does allow for a choice in variable situations.

It is important to teach the patient that time should be spent on activities that are important to him/her, and that time should be organized in a satisfying, productive manner. People with MS need to identify what is important to them and must not lose track of what they are living for.

Lifetime goals become important, since taking control of ones life is connected to these major goals. Time should not be spent on activities that are of no importance.

People have to learn to say "No," an important word in time management. Sometimes the "No" is to the person himself rather than only to others. This may be especially hard for the person with MS, who often already feels guilty about not contributing what s/he feels to be a fair share.

Since no one can do everything, saying "No" may prevent uncomfortable situations with co-workers, family, and friends. It also leads to the ability to say "Yes" to things that matter. It leads to more control over time, and to more time to pursue important goals.

ENERGY CONSERVATION PRINCIPLES

MS usually results in a state of diminished energy. Thus to be effective one must be efficient and conserve as much energy as possible. Following are several techniques which, when employed, can result in more energy and its better use.

1. Balance activity with rest—remember that "rest" means doing nothing at all.
2. Plan ahead
3. Prioritize
4. Pace appropriately
5. Learn activity tolerance

TECHNOLOGICAL DEVICES

Advanced technology can be adapted for many people with disabilities. Therapists therefore need to learn about electronic and technical aids and to keep up with advances in these areas. Historically, "therapeutic occupation" has focused on meaningful tools, trades, and activities. In the 1800s, farming, weaving, and woodcrafting were necessary to daily life and valued in society. In the 1900s, computers, remote controls, and electronic banking are a part of daily life. By becoming involved with technology, occupational therapists can offer their patients therapeutic activity with technological "tools," while providing meaningful and valued access to daily activities.

Adapted Computer Access

Adapted computer access can compensate for many of the physical losses that occur in MS. Computer use has become increasingly easy, as user-friendly, menu-driven programs have become the norm. Computers are typically operated by pressing keys on a keyboard and looking at a display monitor. Any deviation from this falls into the category of an "adaptation." For example, making the keyboard keys larger is an adaptation that makes the computer "accessible," or usable, by a person with hand incoordination.

Adapted computer access devices fall into two categories, those that relate to the inputting of information and those that allow its output to be received. Both input and output adaptations must be appropriate for the user's physical and cognitive abilities. The occupational therapist is well suited to match the disabled user's needs to the most appropriately configured computer system; this is much like adapting any tool to a patient's particular need to allow them to achieve greater independence.

Informing the computer that it is ready to be utilized is the first "input" problem for the user. Power switches may be located almost anywhere, but are frequently on the backs or sides of the computer, monitor, and printer. A simple adaptation is to plug all the system components into a multiple outlet surge protector with a single "on" switch. The outlet strip can then be positioned so that a disabled user can activate it. If operating the switch is too difficult, a remote control switch can be provided.

The two ways to adaptively input information to a computer are direct selection of keys and scanning methods. Direct selection is always preferred because it is much faster than scanning, and direct selection modes should be exhausted before considering a scanning technique.

Direct Selection

Direct selection refers to individual keys being chosen and activated by the user. Methods include finger-pointing, headstick, mouthstick, and optical headpointer. Individual characters may be selected, or a particular key may have "memory" of an entire command sequence (similar to an auto-dial memory feature on the telephone). With that feature the total number of individual key activations can be reduced.

A keyguard is a plastic cover placed over the keyboard with cutout openings over each key (Fig. 3.1). It allows the hand to rest or slide over the keyboard without hitting adjacent, erroneous keys. This approach works well for the "one-two" fingered typist (Columbus system). Because the lettering on the keys may be hard to see with the keyguard in place, enlarged key symbols are helpful. A keyguard is also cumbersome and slow for the patient who is able to use both hands semi-appropriately.

Enlarged key symbols can be used to assist the visually impaired or a person who is totally unfamiliar with keyboard layouts. These improve body positioning, reduce eyestrain, and improve efficiency in locating the desired key.

Enlarged keyboards (Fig. 3.2), which have larger dimensions than the standard keyboard, allow a person with impaired coordination to accurately select the keys. They are usually fabricated from membrane

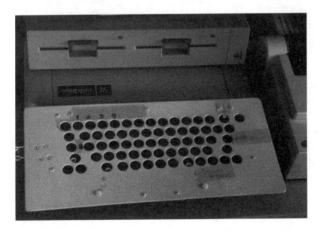

FIGURE 3.1.
Adapted keyguard.

keypads. Several models of enlarged keyboards are commercially available, and have user-friendly customizing capabilities. A particularly versatile expanded keyboard for users with MS is the Unicorn Expanded Keyboard by Unicorn Engineering.

Miniature keyboards are reduced in size (i.e., 7 1/2" x 4 1/2") for those with a very limited range of movement. They require good movement accuracy, and are usually operated by a stylus.

Custom keyboards are physically altered or programmed differently than a standard keyboard. These are necessary only when no commercial product fits the user's needs, as they are quite costly to build.

Virtual keyboards represent a standard keyboard in a graphic image on the screen display. A cursor is moved by mouse or by a head or eye movement detection system. Characters are entered as if the standard keyboard was in use.

Scanning Methods

Scanning is much slower and should be considered only when no method of direct selection is effective. Scanning techniques allow total access to a computer system for individuals who cannot effectively use direct selection.

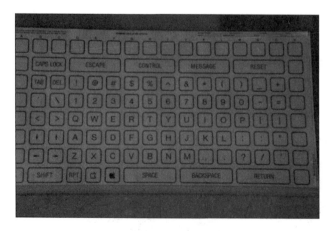

FIGURE 3.2. Keyboards may be enlarged, as shown here, and/or expanded to fit the circumstances of each disability.

The concept of *scanning* has become more familiar with the advent of electronic, digital display radios, often used in automobiles. In one method of scanning access to a computer, keys are represented in an array near the bottom of the computer screen. The array is electronically *scanned* by a cursor movement, moving (blinking) each character in the line-up. When the cursor is blinking on the desired character, a switch is activated by the user, thereby relaying the information to the computer as if that key had been depressed. The scanning is said to be "transparent" to the computer's operation, i.e., the computer acts as if a keyboard input had been received.

Scanning may be *auditory* rather than visual, with a synthesized voice output used to announce the array. When the desired character or command is announced, the user activates a switch to send that character or command to the computer.

A variety of switch mechanisms can work with scanning selection methods. It takes considerable skill to match the most appropriate body site and motion to the proper switch and switch placement, e.g., a lever switch mounted on the inside of a wheelchair armrest to be activated by humeral abduction, or a chin switch mounted on gooseneck pipe affixed to a desktop.

The information generated by the computer must be in a form usable to the computer operator. The usual small letters on a computer screen may not be practical for the MS patient with visual problems. Several adaptations are available for changing the output, including a larger display on the screen, achieved by software, a larger monitor, magnification, closed-circuit TV enlargement, or speech output-which refers to the computer "saying" what is on the screen or what key has been depressed. These may be achieved by software and the talking Unicorn Expanded Keyboard.

In evaluating an individual for computer use, a standard, thorough occupational therapy examination should include an evaluation of motor, sensory, and cognitive function, a social and physical environmental analysis, as well as an analysis of self-care, productive pursuits, visual acuity, and leisure pursuits.

The treatment plan should not only include traditional approaches, but also be directed toward therapeutic activity. A detailed analysis should be made of each patient's interest level, the availability of a computer, past computer experience, communication skills, hand coordination, the desire to learn, benefits of accessing electronic "communities," and cognition. As with any therapeutic modality, goal setting is essential. The treatment plan includes orientation, evaluation, training, and treatment activities.

As each individual is being evaluated for computer use, proper software selection is essential to meet treatment goals. Factors to consider include ease of use ("friendliness," clarity of instructions, one step versus multiple step responses), quality and size of visuals and graphics, adaptability of programs, feedback systems, and whether the software fits the intended purpose.

Environmental Control

Another important aspect of modern technology that can greatly enhance the quality of life of individuals with MS is that of "environmental control" which refers to an individual's capability to control his/her environment via remote control. Such controls have become commonplace for garage door openers and televisions, and special applications can be had at relatively low cost.

The control switch can be any of some 200 currently available in the rehabilitation technology market (Fig. 3.3). The occupational thera-

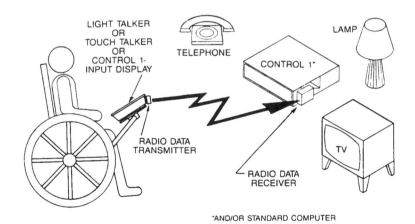

Figure 3.3. Example of wireless data system.

pist is instrumental in assessing the point of body control that will most reliably allow the patient to consistently and voluntarily activate the switching device, and to determine the type of switch needed. Several control sites and several switch types may need to be evaluated before finding the most efficient ones. Practice over time with the switch may improve efficiency; this should be considered when making the final recommendation. Environmental control units are composed of determined switch plugs, which vary from a device designed to operate a single electrical appliance to centralized, multidevice units and computer-based systems.

Many types of appliances may be controlled by environmental control units, including lamps, radio, television, climate control (furnace, air conditioner, fan, humidifier, dehumidifier), telephone, electric hospital bed controls, call buttons, small appliances (coffee maker, tape player, stereo system), electric track drapes, and electric doors and locks. The greater the mobility impairment, the greater positive impact the ability to control the environment can have for the patient. As with any type of adaptive equipment, the individual may at first feel more "disabled" by needing it. Education and familiarity with the equipment can allow a return to independence for the individual, the development of a greater sense of control, and less dependence on others to do everyday tasks.

Costs for environmental controls and funding for the purchase of these units is highly variable. It is always worth trying to apply for insurance reimbursement based on the patient's increased ability to summon emergency help and to reduce costs for the attendant care that would otherwise be needed for these tasks.

Third-party payors should consistently be confronted with requests for these type of devices. Even if they are rejected, hopefully with time they will realize the need for these devices. If therapists do not submit requests due to the preconceived idea that they will be rejected, the insurers will never be made aware that the need exists.

Another possible source of funding is the local vocational rehabilitation agency. In some states, "homemaker" is a vocational category, and a case can be made that an environmental control device will make an individual more independent in the home.

Any individual who acquires an environmental control device must be properly trained in its use. In addition, the device, control switch, switch mounting or positioning may need customization. Follow-up to adjust the system's parameters is necessary as the patient gains efficiency with the unit.

DRIVING

The ability to drive is intimately tied to our society's concepts of freedom and independence. For the adult who must stop driving due to a disability, the loss is more than just that of mobility—it is a loss of the freedom to decide when and where to go. Needing to ask others for rides and waiting incessantly to be picked up and delivered is the antithesis of independence. The experience is likened to being treated like baggage! A loss of self-esteem and dignity is therefore inevitable when the decision is made that a person may no longer drive.

The occupational therapist plays an important role in helping the rehabilitation team determine whether continued driving is feasible. The occupational therapist has not only the ability to assess some of the skills related to driving, but also the perspective of what impact the ability to drive, or its loss, will have on an individual's ability to carry out daily living tasks. This perspective allows the occupational therapist to plan interventions that will promote both maximum independence, and maximum adaptation to changes in previously valued roles.

Any credible intervention begins with a thorough assessment. It is worthwhile to locate and develop communication with a rehabilitative center that offers specialized driver assessments. These vary widely in scope, and may be done by an occupational therapist, physical therapist, driving instructor, or a vocational counselor. The best assessments will include (1) a test of physical, visual, and cognitive function (attention span, distractibility, memory, judgement); (2) computer-rated driving simulation, with or without automobile adaptations; and (3) a road test.

An assessment that neglects one or two of these areas will miss important skill information. MS patients with minor physical disability, but substantial cognitive impairment, may pass simple road tests done in parking lots with pylons, but be dangerously unsafe drivers when faced with the cognitive and attentional demands of driving in traffic. It is extremely important that the referring health care center provide as much background on the patient as possible to the specialized driving assessment facility. This allows for a better understanding of the reasons for the referral and alerts the examiners to potential skill and deficits.

Depending upon the level of physical impairment, it may be relatively simple to regain driving independence. For lower extremity weakness, spasticity, or incoordination, hand controls may be a feasible alternative. For the one-handed driver, a steering knob will improve efficiency and control in steering. Van and automobile wheelchair lifts can be installed by qualified companies to improve mobility.

States vary on the reporting of results from specialized driving assessments. Some automatically report results to the state bureau of motor vehicles, while others do not release information unless the patient has signed a release. Physicians can often override the patient's desire for privacy of their driving assessment performance and have the scores reported, and should do so if they believe that the patient's driving could endanger his/her life or that of others. Check with a rehabilitation facility providing specialized driver assessments in your state to stay apprised of the current policies.

STRESS AND RELAXATION

Many behavioral adjustments occur in response to the fast pace and pressure of modern life. Change, whether good or bad is always a stressor, and life events such as accidents, divorce, death, changing jobs, and moving are major stressors.

Living with MS means change and stress, not only for the person with MS but also for friends and family. Chronic disability leads to stressors that include

1. Role conflicts
2. Unpredictability
3. Loss of both emotional and physical control
4. The stress of dealing with a chronic disease on a day to day basis

Stress depletes an individual both emotionally and physically and adds to fatigue. Everyone, with or without MS, can benefit from stress reduction skills and relaxation techniques.

Stress management and relaxation should be taught as part of a total wellness approach, which includes both proper exercise and nutrition. Stress management often fits well with individual, group, or family counseling.

Medical evidence shows no clear, specific evidence that stress is a causative factor in MS. However, as in all neurological disease, stress does exacerbate the symptoms of the disease process. Thus patients perform poorly when under stress. Stress education should focus on

- Identifying causes of stress
- Recognizing physical signs of stress
- Exercise and stress reduction techniques
- Nutrition
- Relaxation
- Personal planning

The following questions should be addressed with the patient during the initial evaluation:

1. What is the patient's attitude toward health-directed changes in lifestyle?
2. Is the patient willing to take some responsibility for change? Does s/he generally take an active role in problem-solving or is s/he a passive player?
3. Does s/he agree that learning relaxation requires a commitment to practice each day in a quiet, undisturbed location?

After these questions are addressed, an objective assessment should evaluate the following factors:

1. Physical status—complaints of pain, functional abilities, diet, exercise
2. Mental status—self-perception of emotional and intellectual styles, supports and coping behavior time management techniques; much of this information can be obtained by the psychologists working with the individual
3. Social status—living situation, work and family relationship issues

4. Vocational/avocational—current interests, past interests, typical day's schedule.

It is important that the rehabilitation professional address mental health issues when appropriate. One must understand what causes stress in order to deal with it. Stress can include anything from breaking a fingernail to driving in heavy traffic to significant family problems. The patient should be asked to keep a diary of stressful events over a period of 1–2 weeks or try to recall what caused stress during a single week.

Physical symptoms are warnings that stress is becoming a significant problem. It is important that patients be taught to listen to their bodies and adjust their lifestyles accordingly. Some common stress-related changes include increases in fatigue and/or spasticity, sleeplessness, nightmares, muscle tightening in the neck and shoulder area, and headaches.

An exercise program for the MS patient should utilize stress-reduction techniques that include the following:

1. Learning to accept what cannot be changed
2. Talking out worries and frustrations
3. Avoiding self-medication and the use of alcohol, caffeine, or nicotine
4. Balancing work and recreation
5. Getting adequate amounts of sleep
6. Taking one thing at a time, learning to prioritize and manage time.

The purpose of relaxation is to consciously dampen physical processes through manipulation of cortical influences. This is based on the belief that the mind influences the body and the body influences the mind. Patients need to understand what happens physiologically as one relaxes—muscle tension decreases, which can help reduce spasticity, the heart and respiratory rates slow, and mental attention shifts, helping to increase concentration.

Relaxation techniques vary from the most concrete (tense-relax, deep breathing) to moderately concrete (imagining a familiar scene) to abstract (imagery, visualization). Patients should be encouraged to choose what seems most enjoyable and helpful for them.

It is helpful to use a flow sheet to record day to day responses (Fig. 3.4) The use of biofeedback can give an objective grading system. Heart rate, respiratory rate, blood pressure, or even facial expression, can be used as a measure of relaxation. Subjective responses should also be recorded. The goal of stress management and relaxation is to change self-defeating attitudes in order to facilitate good, healthy adjustments to a chronic illness.

ACTIVITIES OF DAILY LIVING

Activities of daily living (ADL) can be made easier when the occupational therapist helps the patient to learn different ways to accomplish tasks, and teaches him/her how to use specific pieces of adaptive equipment. The therapist may also recommend that the environment be rearranged so as not to present barriers to activities. The patient's level of disability may change at any time, and such recommendations will need to be modified when this occurs.

The selection of the proper adaptive device and technique requires a comprehensive approach that includes an evaluation of the patient's needs, priorities, and motivation to use devices. The goals are to increase the level of independence, restore a specific function, maintain that function, and to perform an activity as efficiently as possible to allow time and energy for other activities.

The selection of adaptations or compensatory techniques is based on the patient's symptoms and how they interfere with skills or performances. Multiple factors or symptoms often interact to decrease performance capability.

The therapist needs to involve the patient in the process of determining ADL adaptations and to give the patient control over the choice of adaptations. S/he must also help the patient work through psychological barriers against adaptive devices and altered techniques. For some individuals, using a different method and different device means "handicapped" and further emphasizes the realism of disability. These individuals insist on using the same old method and fighting even when it no longer works for them. The therapist needs to point out the advantages of changing, e.g., a new method or device saves

Date	Heart Rate		Blood Pressure		Respirations per Minute		Comments
	Pre	Post	Pre	Post	Pre	Post	

RIVERSIDE MEDICAL CENTER
Occupational Therapy Department
RELAXATION RESPONSE RECORD

FIGURE 3.4. Flow sheet to record responses during relaxation exercise.

energy that can be used for enjoyable tasks. Also, a trial period should be encouraged to let the patient know they still have the right to decide and control what method or device will eventually be used.

On the other end of the spectrum, there is the patient that wants all available equipment and may seem over-eager to learn new methods. The therapist needs to seek out the motivation for this need. Is it poor self-esteem, or is there secondary gain and attention from being handicapped? The patient is often not even attuned to his/her needs. The therapist must help the patient strike a balance and look at priorities, allowing the choice of what is essential for independence.

All of the above can be complicated by cognitive deficits affecting judgment and new learning. The patient may deny problems or refuse adaptive equipment but have documented difficulties that affect safety. The family should then become involved through family conferences and make recommendations for change. In more severe safety situations, social services should be involved to ensure adult protection. Videotaping performance to use as a teaching tool and to instill more patient insight may also be helpful.

The first step in evaluating the patient is to discuss what are his/her everyday activities and what problems are encountered. Ideally, this would be followed by a home or worksite visit, to find solutions to problems or alternative ways of doing things. A sketch, with measurements, should be made of the living or work area (Fig. 3.5). This can be immensely helpful in the future if new problems arise, at which time making changes in the environment, using it differently, or introducing a large piece of durable medical equipment, can be considered without making a return visit.

For example, if careful measurements are taken of all the doorways in the home, the placement of the bathroom fixtures, and the placement of kitchen appliances, the occupational therapist can use this information later when the patient might be considering a wheelchair. The answers to the following questions will be obvious: Will the wheelchair be able to enter all the rooms or will the doorways need to be widened? Will the patient be able to use the bathroom sink or will the kitchen sink be more accessible, if a lowered mirror and shelf to hold grooming supplies are added? Which hot water and drainage pipes should be wrapped with insulation to prevent burns to the legs? Does the refrigerator door open in the right direction to per-

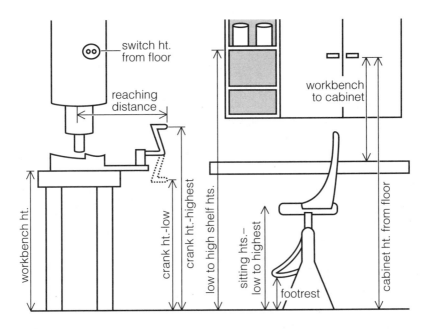

FIGURE 3.5. Schematic of living or work area.

mit easy access from a wheelchair. Will a commode fit at the bedside to avoid time-consuming nighttime transfers from the bed to the wheelchair into the bathroom and onto the toilet. Is there room for that commode to fit over the toilet or parallel to the tub?

When making site visits it is better to err on the side of taking too many measurements. Adaptive equipment for self-care, homemaking, and communication includes many devices that have proven to be helpful in dealing with the wide range of disabilities experienced by people with MS. Because this range is so wide, a discussion of each type of equipment and how it can be used is beyond the scope of this book. This shared challenge is usually a learning experience for both the patient and therapist. The tables presented in the following sections summarize adaptive devices and techniques for a number of activities of daily living. The reader is also referred to the many catalogs of adaptive devices now available (see Appendix).

Self-Care

BATHING

The patient with minimal lower extremity weakness or balance problems should find that a rubber bath mat, a vertical grab bar where s/he enters the tub, and a diagonal grab bar on the long wall are sufficient for safety (Fig. 3.6). Any patient who is in danger of falling while getting into or out of the tub should take a seated shower using a transfer tub bench and an extension shower hose. Patients with good stability and sliding transfer skills may use a water-powered chair lift. A Hoyer® or Trans-Aid® bath attachment can be used to transfer a patient in a sling from a wheelchair into the tub using an inflatable cushion behind his/her head. Inflatable shampoo basins are available for the bedbound patient, and Trans-Aid® makes a vinyl tub for use in bed that is filled and drained by a hose that can be attached to any faucet. Hot baths or showers that could cause the body core temperature to rise must be avoided, as heat exacerbates many of the symptoms of MS. Table 3.1 lists adaptive devices and techniques of use during bathing.

TOILETING

Drop-arms and wheels are important options to consider when a commode becomes necessary. Drop-arms may become necessary for sliding transfers, and a commode on wheels may be able to pass through very narrow (20") bathroom doorways. The most commonly needed toilet adaptations are an armrest support (attached to the toilet or the wall) and a raised toilet seat. A seat with a front cutout will make catheterization easier and provide more room for toileting.

GROOMING

Patients with tremor or ataxia have the most difficulty with grooming. One-pound wrist weights help some patients, and holding the arms close to the chest provides some stabilization when using an electric razor or toothbrush.

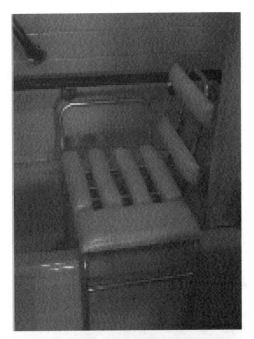

FIGURE **3.6.** Bathing aids. **A:** Transfer tub bench. **B:** Standard chair lift for bathing (Hoyer®).

A

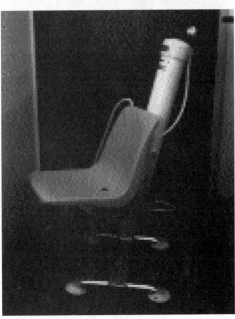

B

TABLE 3.1 BATHING

ADAPTIVE DEVICE OR TECHNIQUE	SYMPTOMS			
	TREMOR	WEAKNESS	FATIGUE	SENSATION
Use of tub bench in bath or shower (feet should touch floor for stability)	X	X	X	
Hand-held shower	May be difficult to handle	X		
Long bath sponge to reach arms and legs	X	X	X	
Use of bath thermometer to gauge temperature				X
Grab bars (never use soap dish or towel racks, as these can pull out of wall)	X	X	X	
Bath mitt eliminates searching for dropped soap	X	X	X	X Soap may easily slip due to poor sensation
Avoid hot water, is it increases fatigue and increases body temperature			X	X Turn down water heater to eliminate chance of burn
Organize shampoo, soap, etc., and keep within reach		X	X	
Build up toothbrush, comb, brush		X		
Transfer tub bench can be used when unable to step over tub	X	X		
Hydraulic lift can be used if patient is dependent in transfers		X Usually severe weakness		

DRESSING

Whenever possible the patient should dress in easy to wear styles and slip-on shoes. The Swedish Stocking Aid is helpful in putting on socks and a reacher or long shoe horn assists with shoes. Because using pantyhose is nearly impossible for women with severe lower extremity weakness and some truncal or upper extremity weakness, alternatives such as longer skirts and knee-high stockings should be considered. The button on a shirt cuff can be managed by (1) using a button-aid, (2) moving the button over to enlarge the cuff opening, (3) re-sewing the button on with elastic, or (4) replacing the button closure with Velcro. Table 3.2 lists adaptive devices and techniques of use while dressing.

EATING

When weakness makes it difficult for the patient to hold silverware, try the Vertical Palm® or Horizontal Palm Self-Handle Utensils®. The Splint with Utensil Holder offers wrist support. The T-shaped handle of the Lightweight Plastic Handle Mug® can slip between the fingers and anchor the mug in a weak grasp.

Ataxia and tremors pose a major problem for eating. Wrist weights, weighted utensils, and holding the arms close to the body may help. Plastic glasses with lids and openings for straws are good for cold drinks. The Vac-U-Flow® cup will hold hot coffee, has a built-in nipple, and cannot spill more than one drop (the fluid must be sucked out). The cup should be placed in a heat-resistant holder, such as foam or thick terry cloth. Dycem or clamps should stabilize the plate. Table 3.3 lists adaptive devices and techniques of use while eating.

HOMEMAKING

After you have determined how much homemaking your patient will actually be doing, and how much can reasonably be shared with others, help him/her look for ways to organize the tasks and space, discuss labor saving devices and appliances, and teach safety techniques.

TABLE 3.2 DRESSING

ADAPTIVE DEVICE OR TECHNIQUE	SYMPTOMS			
	TREMOR	WEAKNESS	FATIGUE	SENSATION
Sit while dressing		X	X	
Dress weaker side first		X	X	
If legs are weak, use sock aid, long reacher long shoehorn, eliminates need to pick up weak leg to dress feet and legs		X	X	
Slip-on shoes are easier than tie shoes	X	X	X	
Use Velcro for closure on pants, skirts, shirts	X	X		X
Wear pullover tops	X	X		X
Sew cuff buttons on with elastic thread	X	X		X
Use buttonhook for small buttons	Can use if tremor is not pronounced	X		X
Lower closet bar for clothes		X		
Wear adapted clothes, i.e., wrap-around skirts, mid-calf skirts that cover knees when seated, etc.		X		

TABLE 3.3 EATING

| ADAPTIVE DEVICE OR TECHNIQUE | SYMPTOMS | | | |
	TREMOR	WEAKNESS	FATIGUE	SENSATION
Use of plate guard	X	Good for hemiplegia		
Weighted utensils	X	Contraindicated	Contraindicated	
Insulated mugs with lid	X Some mugs come weighted	X	X	X
Rocker knife for cutting		Good for one-handed cutting		
Placing plate or cup on a nonslick surface, i.e., textured placement or damp wash-cloth	X			
Build up eating utensils		X		X
Sip liquids from a long straw	X	X		
Hold arms close to torso or set elbows on table to stabilize	X			
Use both hands to hold cup or glass	X	X		
Adapted cervical collar to stabilize head	X			
Universal cuff to hold utensils		X		

97

MEAL PREPARATION

Kitchen utensils can be organized according to their usage and where they will be used. The easy-to-reach places will be between shoulder and knee height, about 6" short of arm's length. Storage can be maximized by using lazy-Susans, pull-out platforms on counters, and pegboards. Seldom-used items should be stored in hard-to-reach places. Since it is less tiring to work while seated, look for ways to provide a lowered workspace such as with a fold-down table that is hinged to the wall at an appropriate height. A cart on casters will be helpful in gathering the utensils and foodstuffs needed to prepare a meal, and in clearing the table.

Faucets that are difficult to reach can be fitted with extensions or replaced by easier to manage paddle handles. Fortunately, there are numerous devices to aid the patient in opening modern containers. One of the most clever is a carton opener from Sweden that makes it possible to open cardboard milk or juice containers with one hand.

Countertop appliances such as coffeemakers and convection or microwave ovens may be easier and safer to use than larger built-in appliances. Several important safety techniques are as follows:

- Use a flint lighter (available at camping stores) to light a gas stove
- Never lift hot liquids across the body (food can be boiled in a steamer or deep-fry basket, and hot liquid can be removed with a ladle or a baster)
- Use long utensils when cooking
- Stabilize mixing bowls and cutting boards when in use
- Use heat-resistant mitts when removing food from the oven.

Table 3.4 lists adaptive devices and techniques of use while working in the kitchen.

HOUSECLEANING

From a seated position, a 30"-handle makes it easier to use a broom, dustpan, or self-wringing mop. Small, lightweight vacuum cleaners are easier to use than standard sized models. Table 3.5 lists adaptive devices and techniques of use when cleaning.

TABLE 3.4 HOMEMAKING/KITCHEN

ADAPTIVE DEVICE OR TECHNIQUE	SYMPTOMS			
	TREMOR	WEAKNESS	FATIGUE	SENSATION
Store items within easy reach in standing or sitting positions		X	X	
Utilize slide-out drawers, cake pan dividers, and other kitchen organizers		X	X	
Sit while preparing meals, washing dishes, etc.		X	X	
Use microwave to eliminate extra dish-washing and save time	X Less chance of burns—microwave is cool	X	X	X
Use wheeled utility cart to carry items and save steps		X	X	
Use wall-hung or under-counter jar opener		X		X
Use food processor to eliminate chopping/grating by hand	X Decreases chance of cutting self with hand-held knife	X	X	X
Slide objects instead of carrying them	X	X	X	
Use unbreakable dishes	X	X		X

99

TABLE 3.4 (CONTINUED)

ADAPTIVE DEVICE OR TECHNIQUE	SYMPTOMS			
	TREMOR	WEAKNESS	FATIGUE	SENSATION
Use electric skillet to reduce transferring on/off range and in/out of oven	X	X	X	X
Use crock pot			X Start meal in AM—more energy/ time	
Use pots/pans with large or double handles	X	X	X	X
Bring all items to one place before starting meal preparations			X Eliminates extra steps	
Use long oven mitts, prevents forearms from touch hot sides of oven	X	X		X
Build up handles on mixing spoons, forks, etc.		X Increases grasp		
Select foods requiring minimal preparation, i.e., frozen, canned, packaged mixes	X	X	X	
Line baking pans with foil to minimize cleaning; soak pots/pans to eliminate scrubbing			X	
Boil food in a steamer or deep fry basket; remove hot liquid and ladle food from pot	X	X		
Use flint lighter to light gas stove	X	X		X

100

TABLE 3.5 CLEANING

	SYMPTOMS			
ADAPTIVE DEVICE OR TECHNIQUE	TREMOR	WEAKNESS	FATIGUE	SENSATION
Spread tasks out over a period of time			X	
Do heavier chores (e.g., washing floors, shopping) in the morning, when energy is highest			X	
Use of a pail to transport cleaning supplies from room to room will save extra trips		Use spray pump vs aerosol if fingers are weak	X	Use rubber gloves if working with strong chemicals
Use long-handled feather duster or vacuum hose to reach low and high surface		X	X	
Buy clothes with easy-care labels to avoid ironing			X	
Sit while ironing			X	
TOILETING				
Use commode at side of bed to save trips to bathroom at night		X	X	
Can use regular commode with catch pan removed over toilet; gives grab bar support and raises seat height		X		
Indwelling catheter eliminates heavy transfers for patient and caregiver		X	X Decreases fatigue for patient	

LAUNDRY

Front-loading machines are easier than top-loading ones to use from a seated position. An area away from the heat should be found to sort, fold, and hang the clothing, and the advantages of fabrics that do not require ironing should be discussed with the patient.

MOBILITY AIDS OTHER THAN AMBULATION AIDS OR WHEELCHAIRS

Patients whose ambulation is only moderately affected may need only minor changes in the home, such as appropriately placed railings. For those more severely affected, ramps, stairglides, and porch lifts can be used to make most homes or buildings accessible. The recommended ramp incline is a 1" rise for every 10"–12" of length. It may not be possible for the patient to negotiate a steeper incline without assistance, and some motorized scooters cannot handle steeper inclines.

Seat-lift chairs can assist patients with lower extremity weakness, but good balance, to get up from a chair.

When the patient requires maximal assistance, patient lifters such as the Hoyer® or Trans-Aid® make safe transfers possible for both the caregiver and the patient (Fig. 3.6). The Trans-Aid® has two advantages over other patient lifters: it can be lowered to the floor to pick up a patient who has fallen, and the patient does not have to remain seated on the sling, which can be removed or reattached while s/he is seated in a wheelchair.

EMPLOYMENT

Available employment statistics for the MS population of working age indicate that about one third is employed, one third is "retired", and one third is not working. Unemployment rates may reach as high as 75%. Many factors are involved in determining whether someone with MS may work, including (1) decreased mobility, (2) spasticity, (3) incoordination, (4) bowel and bladder disturbances, (5) visual difficulty, (6) fatigue, (7) duration and course of disease, (8) the presence of cognitive dysfunction, (9) work-site characteristics, and (10) flexibility in work schedule.

Psychological Influences

Psychological influences may be as important as employment and physical factors in relation to work. Depression, anxiety, self-esteem, the presence of cognitive dysfunction, and the individual's perception of his/her health status all influence employment decisions. It may be of value to begin vocational counseling soon after the diagnosis is made, starting the process of learning and adapting early in the course of the disease so that necessary changes will be planned rather than suddenly forced on the patient and family.

Even individuals with MS who remain employed are likely to encounter situations related to their MS which hinder their job performance. Many are able to make changes that enable them to continue working, such as eliminating barriers, a flexible work schedule, or having access to physical assistance when needed. Disclosure of the MS diagnosis can open avenues for problem solving, but there may also be negative responses relating to unrealistic anticipation of decreased productivity, increased absenteeism, and instability on the job.

Motivation appears to be the key ingredient to success in continuing to work. The rehabilitation team should make every reasonable effort to facilitate employability, identify each vocational issue, and deal with problems as soon as they develop (Table 3.6).

Range of Services

The occupational therapist is a key member of the team involved in vocational rehabilitation. S/he should be aware of the potential course of the disease, the variety of symptoms that may occur, and the functional effects of these symptoms individually and in combination. The therapist can provide a range of services:

TABLE 3.6 WORK PLACE ADAPTATIONS

ADAPTIVE DEVICE OR TECHNIQUE	SYMPTOMS					
	TREMOR	WEAKNESS	FATIGUE	IMPAIRED SENSATION (FEET?)	IMPAIRED SENSATION	IMPAIRED SENSATION
Make sure surfaces and seating are at proper height		X Especially neck, back, trunk	X	X	X	X
Sit as much as possible	X	X	X	X	X	X
Type or dictate if writing is poor or difficult	X	X	X	X	X	X
Use shoulder rest for phone		X	X	X	X	X
Eliminate need to hold phone, use speaker phone or headphones	X	X	X	X	X	
Use phone with large push-button numbers	X					X
Consolidate trips away from work area		X	X	X	X	X
Build up pens/pencils with foam rubber or commercial pen grips		X			X	
Use keyguard for computer/typewriter keyboard	X				X	X
Use cart or two-wheeler to transport items	X	X	X	X	X	X

104

Accommodation			Unilateral weakness		
Use C-clamps, vices, sturdy clips, clipboards, weights to stabilize items	X		X		
Change location of controls to operate machinery (i.e., convert foot pedals to hand controls or vice versa)	X		X	X	
	X		X		X
Extend handles or build up tool/equipment handles	X		X	X	
Use headstick or mouthstick to substitute for lost function	X		X		
Arrange flexible work schedule	X		X		
Use wheelchair or three-wheeler at work			X		X
Use "handicapped parking permit" and/or park close to entrance			X		X

- Testing and evaluation of work abilities related to a specificjob task
- Assessment of learning abilities and retention of skills
- Evaluation of physical, psychological, and social factors such as work tolerance, habits, and interpersonal qualities
- Job task analysis and training in strategies for adapting to specific work situations
- Recommendations to the employer regarding job accommodations
- Prevocational assessment and training
- Assistance to the person with MS in selecting and achieving alternative job situations

Occupational Evaluation

The occupational therapist should conduct a thorough interview that covers the following areas

1. History of occupational performance related to work, self-care, leisure, and social roles as perceived by the patient, including education, past work experience, and specialized training; identifying present and future vocational goals is essential for developing the occupational therapy treatment plan, and should be discussed thoroughly.
2. Attitudes of the MS patient towards his/her job, employer, supervisor, and coworkers, and perceived attitudes of peers and supervisor towards him/her.
3. Current or anticipated job performance issues as seen by the MS person, solutions attempted to date, and results.

To obtain a complete picture of functional abilities, evaluation by the therapist should utilize the following standardized and nonstandardized evaluations:

Daily life tasks: level of independence in self-care, including use of a public restroom or managing in a cafeteria, transportation to and from the job, and mobility on the job;
Range of motion: Specifically address neck, trunk, or extremity limitations which may interfere with turning the head in all

planes, reaching work surfaces, bending, stooping, or sitting.

Muscle strength and tone: Note spasticity or flaccidity, weakness, or ataxia, and their functional significance with regard to tasks performed or positions requiring standing, sitting without support using both arms simultaneously, lifting, carrying, pushing, pulling.

Hand function and coordination: Dominance, grasp and prehension patterns, ability to perform static, dynamic and multiple manipulations.

Endurance and tolerance: Ability to sustain a position or repeat a motion for an extended period prior to fatigue.

Sensation: Tactile, kinesthetic, visual, auditory impairments, and precautions for all compensatory techniques necessary.

Cognition and perception: Attention, memory, and sequencing.

Organization: Ability to analyze, problem solve, and initiate.

Pertinent information should be obtained about the patient's social and financial status, physical capacities, ambulatory/mobility status, comprehension, and speech and language function. Psychological and cognitive testing may also be helpful.

Upon completion of the evaluations the occupational therapist should summarize all deficit areas and symptoms that interfere with function. S/he should also note the abilities of the individual, which will serve as the foundation for analyzing whether his/her job "fits" the individual, and for creating work site modifications or adaptations to the job.

Objective analysis of the patient's job, utilizing all available sources of information, is of extreme importance. First, determine functional job requirements, i.e., tasks which make up the job and anticipated job duties. Obtain a written job description from the employer. Contact the employer or supervisor to clarify any questions about the job description. Then review the job description with the patient to confirm all information and expand on areas of concern. Discuss the following:

- Job duties and responsibilities
- Job components (specific tasks which make up the job)
- Work schedule and breaks

- Equipment and/or tools operated
- Positional requirements: time spent standing, walking, and sitting, twisting crawling, stooping, kneeling, climbing
- Environmental factors: heat, humidity, noise, parking facilities, and distances traveled on the job
- Physical demands: lifting (type of object and frequency, intensity, duration), pushing/pulling (same as above), carrying (type and weight of object and distance), reaching (above, at, and below shoulder height)
- Mental requirements and intellectual demands of the job
- Any other information the patient feels is pertinent to successful performance.

Job Site Visit

If further clarification is needed, a job site visit may be warranted. A comprehensive resource that can be utilized as a format for conducting the job site evaluation is form R-32, used in Worker's Compensation cases. Permission of the employer and the patient is necessary prior to the site visit. When contacting the employer, the therapist should state the purpose of the visit, estimate approximately how much time will be needed, who will need to be involved, and the exact situations the therapist wishes to observe and/or evaluate. In conjunction with the employer, consideration should be given to whether observation of the patient performing the actual work tasks during the site visit would be beneficial; observing the patient directly may be the best way to identify problems and develop modifications of task performance. An employer may more freely reveal behavioral or attitudinal biases in the absence of the worker. What initially appears to be an MS symptom-related problem may instead be a relationship or communication issue. Each situation must be evaluated individually for maximum benefit from performing the job.

When performing the job site evaluation, timeliness, attention to the agenda, and professionalism will be appreciated. For efficiency, the therapist should prepare a list of tasks to observe, work areas to assess, and a list of questions to ask, based on the job description and subjective information previously obtained.

Preparation for the site visit also includes the therapist's preparation of "tools" needed:
- Notepad and pen/pencil
- Copy of the job description
- Tape measure
- Camera or video camera, video film, extra batteries/power source for camera/video
- Dimensions of wheelchair or 3-wheeler if used by the patient on the job, including device height, width, and turning radius

The job site evaluation begins with an evaluation of the physical environment. Since impaired mobility is a major unemployment factor in MS accessibility must be carefully evaluated including

- Parking (distance from entrances)
- Curbs, stairs, ramps elevators
- Doorways (width, threshold obstacles, method, and direction of operation of doors)
- Floor coverings and traffic patterns
- Distances traveled from the usual employee entrance to the work station, between multiple work stations, and from bat rooms/break room to work station.

The second area of evaluation is the "work station," the location(s) where any and all job tasks are performed, where materials are stored, or where equipment is operated. For the auto worker, this may be the assembly line, for the software engineer, the cubicles containing computer hardware and software. Accurate measurements need to be taken of work surface heights in all common positions (sitting, standing, crouching, etc.) and reaching distances (surface to storage, equipment controls, ortho switches).

If possible, the therapist should observe the patient performing tasks representative of the job's most difficult components, and analyze the critical demands of each task with regard to static and dynamic physical requirements of strength, endurance, manipulation, dexterity, position changes, speed, frequency, and duration of repetitive motions. Photographing or videotaping these representative tasks provides an opportunity to later analyze details of the job, tools, equipment, and work site, and acts as a reference when designing specific job modifications.

In summary, job accommodation to enable continued employment may include changing the way the job is done (adapting methods, tools, or equipment), changing the mechanics of the job (work position, environment), changing work habits to increase efficiency or by giving up parts of the job through appropriate delegation or asking for help. Communication with the employer/supervisor is a critical element. The employer may offer major accommodations to enable the MS patient to continue at the original job. If not, a job change within the company may be possible.

If it is determined that the person can no longer continue to work, the pursuit of appropriate, meaningful productive activity will become essential, and counseling/formal support may be needed to adjust to both financial and role changes.

The most important element of keeping the MS patient working is communication among the physician, employer, MS patient, occupational therapist, and vocational counselor. The emphasis is to enable the MS patient to make an informed choice on work issues.

4

SPEECH THERAPY

CAROL KLITZKE, M.A., C.C.C./K.L.P., AND
RANDALL T. SCHAPIRO, M.D.

The production of speech is a motor act that involves the vocal tract via movements of the larynx, vocal cords, palate, tongue, lips, and jaw, and is supported by the respiratory system. Many of the movements needed for speech are affected by multiple sclerosis (MS). Demyelination often occurs in the brainstem, cerebellum, and in the connecting tracts in the cerebrum. These lesions, either singly or multiply, can cause speech difficulties in MS that are termed dysarthria.

Weakness, paralysis, incoordination, abnormal tone, and/or changes in rate are common problems. Speech may be rapid and run together, or slow and labored. It may have a weak, breathy, unarticulated sound to it, or a harsh, tight, spastic quality. A hypernasal quality results when the soft palate is affected. Usually there is a combination of difficulties, giving a "mixed dysarthria." Problems range from the very mild, a slight slur, to the severe, when understanding the speech becomes difficult. The speech processes in MS may improve with remissions of the disease and worsen during exacerbations. Fatigue often affects them severely.

EVALUATION

Evaluation of the speech and language system determines which parts are contributing to communication difficulties and is the basis for developing a therapeutic plan. The evaluation assesses the following characteristics:

1. Oral structure and function, including strength, range of motion, rate, and coordination
2. Laryngeal function (voicing), including intensity, speed and coordination of vocal cord movements, and endurance of voice use
3. Intelligibility of communication attempts
4. Language and cognitive abilities
5. Information gathered from the individual and family regarding his/her daily ability to communicate with others, as well as communication needs at home, work, and in social situations.

AFTER THE EVALUATION

After evaluation, realistic decisions and goals must be determined. Although normal speech or improved neuromuscular function are not realistic outcomes, most individuals with MS do not make the best use of function that does remain. Therefore, therapy usually focuses on compensated communication designed to close the gap between the level at which the individual is communicating, and that which is optimally possible given his/her remaining function.

Unfortunately, individuals are often referred for evaluation and therapy only when speech function is seriously impaired, by which time intellectual function may also be diminished. It is helpful to have individuals referred when speech difficulties first appear; learning and retaining techniques that will compensate for reduced neuromuscular function are easier to teach then, and will carry over into times of more severe difficulties.

TECHNIQUES TO IMPROVE SPEECH

The following techniques are used to improve communication; some of these are taught to the MS person, whereas others are taught to significant listeners in his/her environment. None are intended to "cure" the dysarthria—they help to compensate for the condition.

Use of Pauses

Pausing between every one or two words is helpful when the speech is slurred, rapid, and run together. The result of this technique is dramatic, and previously unintelligible sentences will become clear almost immediately. The technique sounds deceptively simple, but many sessions of therapy are required before a person with dysarthria can develop the appropriate technique, even in the most simple contexts. The ability to self-monitor and to be acutely aware of speech behaviors appears to be diminished in many patients, especially if intellectual function has been affected. Also, after many years of speaking without paying particular attention to it, learning and implementing new patterns is difficult.

Exaggeration

Exaggerating articulation means overpronouncing each word and each sound within words. Particular attention is paid to pronouncing all the speech sounds in each work, especially at their end. Because range of motion of the tongue, lips, palate and vocal cords may be reduced, it is common for many speech sounds to be partially pronounced or omitted altogether. Overarticulating slows the speech process and allows time for the articulators to produce the full range of motion needed to make correct, intelligible sounds.

Increasing Voice Volume

Increasing voice volume simply refers to talking at a level that is too loud for a normal central nervous system, but that actually makes dysarthric speech sound closer to normal. It can be difficult for an individual to get the idea of slowing, exaggerating, and pausing, but a simple reminder from the listener to "talk louder" is easier. The point is not just to make the voice louder, as the voice may be adequately audible if someone is listening carefully. Talking more loudly adds more support and energy to the speech system and at the same time forces the individual to slow down, pause more often, and overarticulate without really thinking about anything but talking more loudly. This process is often too energy consuming to use constantly in ongoing conversation, but is useful in situations when the listener cannot understand a specific message.

Echoing the Speaker

With this technique, the listener repeats every word or every two to three words the patient says. First, it must be determined how many syllables and words the MS speaker can comfortably and easily produce on one average breath of air. The listener then practices repeating that number of words. This technique has the advantage of being controlled by the listener, which is useful if cognitive deficits are present. Echoing not only slows down the patient's speech by inserting frequent pauses, but it gives immediate feedback to him/her about what the listener can and cannot understand. This is much better than having an MS individual, who needs to conserve energy, articulate an entire sentence, only to have the listener respond with a "What?"

Yes or No Questions

If speech intelligibility is severely impaired and none of the above techniques work, conversation can be framed by asking questions which are answered with yes, no, or maybe.

Nonverbal Communication

Nonverbal communication techniques include writing; pointing to letters, words, and sentences on printed communication boards or notebooks; and a variety of electronic communication devices. These seldom are effective with the MS population because intact language processes are prerequisite to successfully using nonverbal systems; by the time speech deteriorates to severe unintelligibility, language and cognitive functions are often affected as well.

However, it may help in certain situations to write down several words in large print, and ask the person to point, nod, or look at his/her choice. For example, you might ask "What do you want to drink?" but not understand the verbal response. This is slow and not very effective for long conversations, but can help shorten certain interactions.

SUMMARY

The goal of speech therapy with MS persons is not to cure the problem, or to improve neuromuscular function. It is to help establish a means of communication, that utilizes remaining abilities to their full potential. If possible, work on speech dysfunction should begin at the initial onset of problems. When speech has become so impaired that it is unintelligible, intellectual impairment is often present as well. If such intellectual impairment prevents successful speech therapy, several communication techniques can be taught to enhance communication. Among these is gesturing: a system of hand signs and facial expressions may allow for a surprising amount of communication when verbal function is decreased. Communication boards are slow, but are often sure methods of expression. These range from simple alphabet boards to complex electronic ones, and their cost may run from almost nothing to quite expensive. There are also several augmentative communication devices available that can magnify sound or even produce sound and speech. Computerized speech is an example of this type of process.

An individualized evaluation and treatment plan is obviously important in each situation. Not only the person's neurologic situation but also his/her financial resources become important in this potentially high technology therapy.

5

SWALLOWING THERAPY

CAROL KLITZKE, M.A., C.C.C./K.L.P., AND
RANDALL T. SCHAPIRO, M.D.

As more becomes known about evaluation and management of swallowing problems in MS, dysphagia is being recognized as a substantial problem. Dysphagia may be loosely defined as difficulty with swallowing, although this definition becomes somewhat hazy with the realization that some people are "silent aspirators"—individuals who do not perceive themselves as having difficulty swallowing but can be shown by videofluoroscopy to aspirate. There is controversy about whether to label this "dysphagia," and whether such silent aspiration should be treated if the patient remains asymptomatic.

At this point the controversy remains unresolved. Ongoing studies of silent aspiration are likely to provide the answers in the future, but for the present it is essential that symptomatic swallowing problems be appropriately managed.

The term swallowing refers to the entire process of deglutition, from placement of food into the mouth to its passage through the cricopharyngeal sphincter into the esophagus. This process occurs in four stages:

1. Oral Preparatory: foods are placed in the oral cavity, chewed, manipulated and formed into a bolus.

2. **Oral:** The food bolus is systematically propelled posteriorly by the tongue in a stripping or squeezing motion. The swallowing reflex is triggered at the point of the anterior faucial arches (the folds of skin near the back of the mouth).

3. Pharyngeal: The swallowing reflex triggers without disrupting the bolus movement. This causes four critical events to occur: the soft palate closes the passage to the nasal cavity, pharyngeal peristalsis squeezes the bolus through the pharynx, the larynx elevates and closes at three sphincters (epiglottis, false folds, and true vocal folds), and the cricopharyngeal sphincter relaxes to allow passage of the bolus into the esophagus.

4. Esophageal: The bolus passes through the relaxed cricopharyngeal sphincter and moves through the esophagus to the stomach.

This process occurs through a combination of voluntary and reflexive movements whose interactive nature is not yet fully understood. It is clear, however, that the swallowing reflex cannot be stimulated without the presence of material in the oral cavity and the voluntary movement and sensation that such materials produce.

Dysphagia may result when lesions in the brainstem alter the functioning of the brainstem and cranial nerves. The type of swallowing disorder depends on how many and which cranial nerves are affected. Those which have significant control of the muscles for swallowing include the fifth (trigeminal), seventh (facial), ninth (glossopharyngeal), tenth (vagus), eleventh (spinal accessory), and twelfth (hypoglossal).

The swallowing center in the medulla oblongata of the brainstem organizes and controls the swallowing reflex. This center has two sides, one on each side of the midline, and has a complex organization, an arrangement that protects the swallowing reflex from being completely obliterated. However, the reflex can be so reduced that it becomes nonfunctional for eating purposes.

A delayed swallowing reflex and reduced pharyngeal peristalsis are the most common problems seen in MS patients, probably due to involvement of the spinal accessory nerve. Reduced laryngeal function, which compromises airway protection, and reduced lingual function, are the next most common disorders which result from involvement of the vagus and hypoglossal cranial nerves, respectively. Combinations of these problems occur as well, and they may worsen or change with progression of the disease.

As with many types of neurologic dysphagias, sensation and awareness are frequently reduced in the oral, pharyngeal, and laryngeal areas. This may be the result of lesions which affect the sensory portions of the cranial nerves. In addition to this physiologically reduced sensation, individuals with MS may lack awareness and insight into the existence and effects of their dysphagia. Such reductions in sensation and awareness, for whatever reason, lead to dangerous silent aspiration and its complications, such as recurring pneumonias.

Two problems related to dysphagia in MS are functional dysphagia and the "so what?" response to the diagnosis. In the former, patients report difficulties in swallowing (often that food "sticks" in the throat) but no physical symptoms can be found even on videofluoroscopy. One such patient complained of material sticking during the video, but in fact all substances presented were clearing the pharynx with no difficulties.

Related to this problem is overreaction to and/or misunderstanding of the diagnosis of dysphagia. One patient became very upset and reported to his physician that he had swallowing problems which would require major eating changes when he had been told that his dysphagia was mild and necessitated taking only minor precautions.

Finally, some MS patients respond to information about their dysphagia with "So what, I have MS so it doesn't matter." This is an understandable response, especially for individuals whose symptom onset was sudden. This may mean not intervening if that is what the person wishes, or managing the dysphagia with simple diet texture changes by the caregiver, at least initially, until the patient is able to accept the situation and participate more in its management.

EVALUATION

Swallowing difficulties in individuals with MS are often reported initially by a family member or healthcare staff person, based on mealtime observation or attempts to give oral medications. About 40% of all individuals with dysphagia do not present with obvious signs of swallowing distress such as choking or coughing; this percentage may even be higher when dealing only with the MS population. Silent dysphagics or silent aspirators may, for example, initially present with pneumonia. Initial identification may also be difficult due to a lack of awareness and denial by the individual.

For these reasons, people involved with MS individuals must be observant for of subtle as well as obvious signs of dysphagia. Indications of possible swallowing dysfunction include

- Gurgling sounds in the throat, sneezing, running nose, and sounds of congestion during and after meals
- Spitting or coughing copious amounts of phlegm, especially following meals or snacks
- An inability to "get food down"
- Unexplained nutritional and/or hydration problems
- Unexplained pneumonia
- Frequent throat clearing, or quiet attempts at throat clearing during meals
- Choking or coughing during eating
- Patient's complaints of food getting caught during eating
- A weak, breathy voice and/or cough

Referral for an evaluation of swallowing function is indicated if any of these symptoms are observed.

A possible swallowing dysfunction must be evaluated in the context of the individual's total ability to function. While physicians, nurses, therapists, and family are involved in such evaluation, the specific evaluation of eating/swallowing and nutrition processes are completed by a dietician and by a swallowing therapist (usually a speech pathologist) in conjunction with a radiologist.

The Dietician's Assessment

The dietician first completes a nutritional assessment, which involves making observations in the following categories:

Physical/Anthropometric/Laboratory Assessments

The individual's physical appearance is observed. Does s/he appear wasted and malnourished? Is the hair thin? Are the skin and mucous membranes dry? Weight and height are measured, but do not indicate body composition; skinfold and muscle circumference measures can provide this information. Laboratory measurements of proteins and blood analyses are used to establish nutritional status.

Individual/Family Interviews

These interviews are often the most significant, or in many cases the only, sources of nutritional information. A careful interview should obtain information about the following dietary habits:

- Food preferences and dislikes
- Changes in food preferences, particularly texture changes; an individual may state s/he "prefers" a certain texture, but in fact it is the only texture he can comfortably swallow
- History of swallowing problems
- Presence of allergies
- Typical meal patterns
- Changes in meal patterns or habits
- History of weight fluctuation
- Fluid intake
- Alcohol intake
- Vitamin and mineral supplementation
- Cultural and religious food practices

Mealtime Observations

Some observations are similar to those made by the speech pathologist, but the dietician pays more attention to amounts and type of food consumed. If there are indications of problems with fluid and caloric intake, calorie counts and fluid intake amounts may be monitored for several days. Mealtime evaluation is discussed in detail below.

The Speech Pathologist's Assessment

The speech pathologist's assessment consists of clinical, meal-time, and videofluoroscopic evaluations done in conjunction with a radiologist.

CLINICAL EVALUATION

The clinical evaluation reviews the pertinent history related to swallowing and examines the status of the visible characteristics of oral, pharyngeal, and laryngeal function. This history should include information about the specific symptoms and their duration, general medical status, respiratory status, feeding route (oral, nasogastric, etc.), and what the patient and family do to alleviate the symptoms. Because decreased awareness and sensation of swallowing disorders is common in the MS population, information obtained from primary care-givers is important. Although the family observes difficulties, the patient may deny them and/or be highly inaccurate about their frequency and severity. If awareness and sensation are intact, patients are usually accurate in pointing to the area causing swallowing difficulties.

Examination should then be made of the structure of all visible parts of the eating/swallowing mechanism and the strength, move-ment, range of motion, and accuracy of movements of the jaw, lips, tongue, and soft palate. The structure and function of the pharynx and larynx can be indirectly examined by asking the individual to swallow while the examiner places fingers on the jaw, hyoid bone, and thyroid cartilage areas. If the swallow reflex is present the larynx should rise. This technique can provide a rough idea of whether a swallow reflex is present, whether it feels complete, and if there may be a delay in initiation. The individual is then asked to clear the throat, cough, and vocalize a loud sustained tone, providing information about airway strength and protection. If there is a weak breathy tone and significant air escape, it may be difficult to maintain closure or the airway during the act of swallowing, or to expel material from the airway.

Throughout the clinical evaluation, observations should be made of head positions, body postures, management of oral secretions, and the presence of congested sounds in the chest and airway.

If observation at a mealtime is not possible, various textures of food may be presented at this time. Evaluation is the same as discussed later for mealtime evaluations. However, this situation is somewhat contrived, and may not provide accurate information.

MEALTIME EVALUATION

The mealtime evaluation involves observation of an individual who eats orally during his/her usual mealtime. Observation should be as unobtrusive as possible to allow natural behaviors to occur in a relaxed atmosphere.

Some of the observations made and questions asked should include: How are various food textures removed from eating utensils? Is food material drooled from the mouth? Is food organized and manipulated by the tongue, or does it sit on the tongue with little movement? Is food moved posteriorly in a controlled manner, or is it propelled by tilting the head back? Is food absentmindedly stuffed into mouth and held there without attempts to swallow? Does the individual demonstrate good judgement regarding size of bolus and rate of intake? Is there evidence of unsafe behaviors such as impulsively laughing or talking midswallow? Can the individual demonstrate follow-through on instructions given? Is there coughing or choking during the meal? If so, when and on which substances? Is there evidence of discomfort or pain during swallows? Are there any signs of silent aspiration, such as eyes watering, loss of breath or voice, gurgling sounds from the throat? What does the individual or caregiver do when difficulties occur?

At various times during the meal the patient should be asked "Where do you feel the food?" and instructed to point to the area. It is not necessary to observe an entire meal. The therapist might come and go, and observe for build up of congestion, amounts consumed over time, and fatigue factors near the end of the meal.

VIDEOFLUOROSCOPY

Videofluoroscopy is a radiographic procedure that visualizes the movements involved in swallowing. It is sometimes referred to as a "cookie swallow" or a modified barium swallow and is conducted by a radiologist, speech pathologist, and radiology technician. The individual is given various textures of barium, including a cookie coated with barium paste, to swallow in small amounts. The posterior oral area, pharynx, and upper esophagus are then viewed in the lateral and anterior-posterior positions via radiographic filming.

The study not only determines the presence of aspiration, but more importantly determines the reasons why it occurs, ranging from impaired tongue movement, a delayed swallowing reflex, reduced pharyngeal peristalsis, weak airway closure, cricopharyngeal muscle dysfunction, reduced sensation, and/or functional/behavioral abnormalities.

In addition to these routine procedures, the effects of certain modifications can be observed. For example, the individual may be asked to change head positions, clear the throat or cough hard, pump the tongue more, or report the sensations felt at various points during the study. This information is very helpful in later management.

Information from these evaluations is summarized, and used to develop a plan of management.

MANAGEMENT

The goal of a swallowing management program is to maintain or improve nutritional status while providing safe oral intake (initially) and to facilitate independent eating and swallowing as long a possible. To achieve this goal it is essential that the dysphagia staff, particularly the dietitian and speech pathologist, review the clinical findings and develop a joint care plan.

As mentioned earlier, major challenges with MS individuals may be denial that a problem exists, reduced sensation, an inability to make judgements regarding management techniques, and difficulty recalling and following through independently with such techniques. A program of dysphagia management may be designed as much for the family and caretakers as for the involved individual. It can be very uncomfortable and anxiety producing to eat meals with a family member who frequently chokes and/or gets food lodged in the throat.

Areas which should be considered when helping an individual and caretakers manage dysphagia include modifications of the eating environment, food textures, eating behaviors, neuromuscular movements and/or feeding methods.

Modification of the Eating Environment

If the individual must pay attention to establishing new behaviors during eating, a quiet, nondistracting environment is probably ideal. This can be a real problem of course, because mealtimes are often social times and many people watch TV while eating meals and snacks. Following are some suggestions that can be given to families:

- Take a CPR class to learn the Heimlich maneuver for clearing material blocking the airway.
- Avoid asking the individual with dysphagia open-ended questions during eating. If you must, ask yes/no questions which can be answered with a head nod.
- Tell jokes or funny stories before or after a meal or during swallowing breaks.
- Provide "safe" meal textures (details of texture are in the next section) when watching TV and eating during a social gathering, which will reduce the need for intense concentration on the act of swallowing.
- Look and choose carefully from restaurant menus. Request additional sauce for dry chunky items, and perhaps carry a small amount of Thick-It® (a commercial thickening agent) to mix discretely with thin liquids.

If the patient has a behavioral or functional type of dysphagia, with associated anxiety and a feeling of tightness in the throat, a more distracting environment may actually be beneficial by taking the focus away from the act of swallowing.

Modification of Food Textures

Some food textures may be easier to swallow than others, depending on the site of the dysphagia. This will be determined from the evaluations discussed earlier. For example, if tongue weakness or paralysis is present, thin liquids may not be controlled well and slip into the pharynx before the airway closes, while solid foods might be more difficult to swallow for those with a cricopharyngeal dysfunction.

Modification of diet textures is the management technique which often gives the fastest results with the least active participation of the individual. This is particularly important for those with cognitive deficits. Providing safe diet textures reduces the risk of aspiration or a blocked airway, reduces the need for supervision during eating, and reduces the need to concentrate and make frequent judgements about eating methods. This can be accomplished most easily in a rehabilitation setting. Nutrition Services offer some staged diets, including thin liquids, thick liquids (nectars, tomato juice), thickened liquids (commercial thickening agents and special recipes), puree, mechanical, soft, regular, and combinations of these.

Based on the results of the swallowing evaluation, a dietitian meets with the patient and/or caregiver to match swallowing needs with nutritional needs and food likes and dislikes. This can be particularly challenging with MS patients, because high fiber diets are frequently recommended due to associated bowel problems. Typically such diets include raw vegetables, fruits with skins and seeds, nuts, popcorn, cereals, and rice, which are among the most dangerous foods for an individual who has a delayed swallow reflex and /or reduced airway protection.

Snacks, treats from friends, pitchers of water delivered to rooms, medications, and modification of meals in the real world settings are more difficult to control than meals provided at scheduled times in the rehabilitation setting.

It is a real challenge to modify snacks and meals while taking into consideration food pleasures, nutrition needs, and the limits of an already overtaxed caregiver, and MS individuals who live alone may have inconsistent attendant assistance. It is therefore essential to provide specific verbal and written information, including recipes; it is not sufficient to verbally recommend the use of thickening liquids, or that all foods be prepared for soft texture.

Following are some suggestions for individuals who require thickened liquids due to delayed swallowing reflex, poor tongue control, or poor airway closure:

- Water will probably be the most difficult item, but also the most missed in the diet. Try using a commercially available thickener, such as Thick-It®, for water and any thin liquids.
- Ice cubes moisten the mouth but melt into liquid before they reach the pharynx. They may create the same problems as water, such as aspiration pneumonia.
- Gelatin and ice cream must be used as thickeners with caution, because they also melt before reaching the pharynx.
- The use of milk, ice cream, and milk shakes as thick beverages may need to be limited, because they mix with saliva and form excess mucous, which is difficult to clear, especially if the coughing and throat clearing function is reduced.
- Try thick fruit beverages such as frappes, blends, shakes, and puree/juice combinations.

Suggestions for individuals who require moist, soft textures due to reduced pharyngeal peristalsis, reduced coughing and throat clearing ability include the following:

- Chop meat and other coarse food materials whenever possible, and moisten it with broth, juices, gravies, or fats. Large, tough meat chunks can easily lodge in the airway, and are perhaps the single most dangerous food substance for an MS individual. The consistency should be dry enough to form a bolus, and moist enough not to crumble.
- Try puffed popcorn snacks rather than regular popcorn.
- Try nut butters in place of dry, chunky, individual nuts if tongue function allows manipulation of sticky items.

Additional dietary suggestions are

- Eat foods that are warmer or colder than body temperature. Foods at body temperature may not sufficiently stimulate chewing and swallowing reactions.
- For psychological reasons, provide a varied diet with as many characteristics of a normal diet as possible. Do not keep individuals on pureed diets indefinitely. Reevaluate at regular intervals.

Although difficulty in swallowing medications is frequently mentioned, simply crushing tablets and mixing with applesauce may solve the problem. Generally, when we think of modifying food substances, we only think of meals and maybe snacks. Left unchecked, difficulty in swallowing medications can lead to many problems.

With reduced pharyngeal peristalsis, pills may remain in the velleculae at the base of the tongue or in the pyriform sinuses above the esophagus. Uncoated pills may then be absorbed in the pharynx, bypassing the liver and therefore changing the amount of the drug absorbed and its effects.

Particular caution must be taken with silent aspirators. Pills may appear "to go down" adequately, because there is no choking or coughing response, but they may enter the pharynx or airway.

Enteric coated pills are meant to dissolve in the intestine, rather than in the stomach. A well-meaning caregiver who observes dysphagia might crush the pill, allowing it to dissolve in the stomach and therefore altering its effect.

Some medications cannot be mixed with a food such as applesauce because the acidity changes the chemistry of the drug. Some microcoated pills can gently be broken apart in water, the water thickened as mentioned above, and then taken safely.

Bulk formers are often recommended for bowel problems. However, they must be taken with large quantities of water. If thin liquids are a problem, thicker liquids can often be substituted.

An excellent resource for dealing with medications and dysphagia is "Alternative Oral Dosage Forms for the Geriatric Patient" by Sandoz Pharmaceuticals, which includes charts of drugs and their various forms, as well as a discussion of dysphagia problems and solutions.

"Modification of eating behaviors" refers to the actions an individual can perform during eating to compensate for dysphagia. If performed consistently they may increase safety and reduce discomfort. Discussed below are several techniques that might be practiced during therapy sessions.

CHANGING HEAD POSITIONS

Tipping the chin downward tends to slow entry of food material, especially thin liquids, into the pharynx. This technique should be suggested if a delayed reflex is present. Tilting the head backward hastens entry of food into the pharynx, and will help if pharyngeal peristalsis or tongue movement is reduced. If a hemiparesis of the pharynx is present, tilting the head to the stronger side, then turning it toward the weaker side, will direct food down the strong side of the pharynx.

If multiple symptoms are present, a head position which alleviates one may exacerbate another. When this occurs the safest position may be head looking forward, with the chin tilted slightly down.

CHANGING SWALLOWING SEQUENCES

Alternating liquid with solid food swallows helps prevent material from sticking in pharyngeal spaces. This should be practiced if pharyngeal peristalsis is reduced. Frequently clearing the throat and dry swallowing will move material away from the airway and out of pharyngeal spaces.

If there is a significant problem with food residue in the pharynx, hold an ice cube and gently rub the tongue to moisten it, spit out excess liquid, and complete extra dry swallows. This allows an individual to clear residue without adding more material.

Individuals with good sensation can feel the residue as "lumps in the throat." They should be cautioned to clear the pharynx before eating additional food. If sensation is reduced, and such material was observed with videofluorscopy, the patient should be told to assume that there is residue.

ALTERING THE SIZE AND FREQUENCY OF MEALS

If the eating process is slow, it may be helpful to reduce the total amount of food taken at each meal, but to increase the number of meals and snacks throughout the day. This approach is safe and may modify the stress of having to take large amounts of food in a short time period to meet nutritional requirements.

Amounts taken per bite or swallow can be reduced by using smaller spoons or special cups with narrowed spouts. Also, repetitive demonstrations of safe amounts can be given during mealtimes. Frequent reminders are given to cut solid food into pieces no larger than a dime—it helps to actually place a dime next to the plate.

PROTECTING THE AIRWAY

Talking and laughing only between swallows, when the pharynx is clear, will reduce the chance that the airway is open while food material passes through the pharynx.

When laryngeal function is reduced, a supraglottic swallow will help to actively protect the airway. This swallow involves holding the breath while swallowing, then releasing it with a hard cough. It usually must be learned by practicing one step at a time, initially without food.

A power swallow is a variation of the supraglottic swallow whose primary function is to help force open the cricopharyngeus muscle at the top of the esophagus. This is useful if the airway protection and pharyngeal function are intact. It involves holding the breath while swallowing very hard. The idea is to create sufficient air pressure above the esophagus to pop open the dysfunctional muscle.

This power swallow was recently tried with an MS patient who complained of significant swallowing difficulty, characterized by a tight, closed-off feeling in the throat. It was apparent during mealtime that he had developed great anxiety related to eating. Swallowing evaluation including videofluoroscopy revealed intact processes except for small amounts of residue just above the esophagus. He quickly learned the power swallow, and was instructed to moisten his mouth and practice dry power swallows before meals. After several days he was eating regular meals using this method. More than anything, it appeared to give him a measure of control over his symptoms and to reduce his anxiety, which perhaps relaxed muscles in the area.

INDIVIDUAL MODIFICATIONS

Many modifications must be developed on an individual basis, depending on food preferences, eating quirks, etc. For example, one MS patient received a gift of cherries. Instead of putting the cherries into his mouth, he held each cherry and chewed around the pit. A simple modification, but an effective and safe one.

The above techniques are effective if they are consistently utilized. However, as was discussed earlier, many individuals with MS have impaired cognitive function. This, coupled with the need to modify life long behaviors, makes change very difficult. To effect change it is essential to keep things as simple as possible. The speech pathologist should therefore identify those few modifications that will have the most impact on swallowing, then have the patient repeatedly practice those behaviors during snacks and/or mealtimes, even if they seem very simple. Ideally, a family member or friend should be instructed similarly so s/he can coach the individual in the home or other settings. If this is not an option, simple, easy to read instructions can be printed on an index card for an individual to refer to during eating.

Those in the individual's living environment should learn the Heimlich maneuver for clearing material blocking the airway.

Modification of the Neuromuscular Processes

Modifying the actual neuromuscular swallowing process of an individual with MS is at best unlikely, given the exacerbations and remissions of the disease, but these processes may change or improve with the use of certain medications.

However, the following exercises and techniques may be used as part of swallowing therapy to stimulate neuromuscular processes and heighten sensation and awareness. These may be most helpful if an individual is neurologically capable of more than s/he is actually doing.

Thermal Stimulation: Thermal stimulation can be used to stimulate delayed reflexes. A long-handled laryngeal mirror is placed in ice water until cold. The back of the mirror head is then repeatedly, and lightly touched to the bottom of the faucial pillars (skin folds near back of mouth). This procedure needs to be done 4-5 four to five times per day for 5–10 minutes for several weeks to a month before results will be seen. However, for some individuals it may heighten sensation awareness just before eating.

Oral Motor Exercises: There are many different types of oral motor exercises, including range of motion and strengthening exercises for lateralization, elevation, and protrusion of the tongue. Exercises for lip closure and strength can also be practiced, which will help form, hold, manipulate, and propel food boluses.

Laryngeal Exercises: If laryngeal incompetence is a problem, exercises can help improve closure. These might consist of vocalizing and/or holding the breath while pushing against resistance.

These exercises and stimulations are not appropriate or beneficial for all MS individuals with dysphagia. In fact they may be useful for only a select few. A major drawback is that to achieve even small improvements they must be performed many times daily over long periods of time. Therefore, the choice of appropriate candidates depends on expected benefits, the ability of an individual to consistently recall and follow through, and/or the presence of a caregiver to assist with follow through.

Modification of Eating Methods

This may be as simple as utilizing different or modified eating utensils, such as smaller, measured spoons or spoons that can help place the food more accurately in the mouth. Using the results of the swallowing evaluation, and assessing the mealtime needs of the individual, occupational therapists can help a great deal with this.

However, in spite of significant modification of food textures, repositioning, therapy, and instruction, some individuals will not be able to obtain sufficient nutrition and/or hydration by oral feeding alone. Those who have reduced responsiveness secondary to poor nutritional status may become more alert and responsive to therapy with the use of a temporary feeding tube.

Such individuals may require a nasogastric tube (a feeding tube placed through the nose, pharynx, and esophagus into the stomach), a regular gastrostomy (a feeding tube is placed into the stomach via a surgical opening in the abdomen), or a percutaneous gastrostomy (PEG). Nasogastric tubes can be a constant source of nose and throat irritation, and therefore long-term use is not recommended. A gastrostomy or PEG allows for adequate nutrition without interfering with oral feeding.

A percutaneous gastrostomy, inserted by using fluoroscopy to view its placement in the stomach, seems to be the least troublesome for patients, if assistance is needed over a long period of time. There seems to be less discomfort, less recovery time, and fewer disruptions to daily activities.

A wide variety of nonoral feeding products are available. The dietician is responsible for determining which products meet the individual's needs.

Combinations of nonoral and oral feeding methods may also be used. For example, a PEG might be utilized to maintain nutrition and adequate hydration over a prolonged period of time. However, oral snacks or very small meals of modified textures may be appropriate for pleasure and enjoyment. A dietician can monitor, adjust, and balance the combination of feeding methods.

SUMMARY

Dysphagia often occurs as a result of MS, but the individual may deny the existence of swallowing problems because of reduced sensation and/or awareness. Family and friends may be the first to notice difficulties. However, if silent aspiration is present, the problem may not be noticed until a problem such as aspiration pneumonia develops. Although dysphagia resulting from MS cannot be cured, a number of management techniques can help. These include modifying the eating environment, food textures, eating behaviors, neuromuscular movements, and feeding methods. Consistently utilized, these management techniques may help continue oral eating as long as possible, in a safe manner which provides adequate nutrition.

Appendix
Suggested Readings

General

DeLisa JA. *Rehabilitation Medicine*. Philadelphia: JB Lippincott, 1988.

Maloney FP, Burks JS, Ringel SP. *Interdisciplinary Rehabilitation of Multiple Sclerosis and Neuromuscular Disorders*. Philadelphia: JB Lippincott, 1985.

Schapiro RT, Van Den Noort S, Scheinberg L. The current management of multiple sclerosis. *Annals NY Acad Sci* 436:425–434, 1984.

Schapiro RT. *Symptom Management in Multiple Sclerosis*. New York: Demos, 1987.

Physical Therapy

American College of Sports Medicine. *Guidelines for Exercise Testing and Prescription*. 3rd Edition. Lea and Feiber, 1986.

Borg G. Psychophysical basis of perceived exertion. *Med Sci Sports Exercise* 14:377–381, 1982.

Chen W, Pierson F, Burnett C. Force-time measurements of knee muscle functions of subjects with multiple sclerosis. *Phys Ther* 67:934–940, 1987.

Freal JE, Kraft GM, Coryell JK. Symptomatic fatigue in multiple sclerosis. *Arch Phys Med Rehab* 65:135–138, 1984.

Gehlsen G, Grigsby S, Winant D. Effects of an aquatic fitness program on the muscular strength and endurance of patients with multiple sclerosis. *Phys Ther* 64:653–657, 1984.

McNeal R. Aquatic therapy. *Phys Ther Forum* 8:13(1–4), 1989.

Noble B. Clinical application of perceived exertion. *Med Sci Sports Exercise* 14:406–411, 1982.

Umphred D. *Neurologic Rehabilitation*. St. Louis: CV Mosby, 1985.

Wilson B. *Wheelchairs: A Prescription Guide*. New York: Demos, 1990.

Occupational Therapy

Dellon AL. *Evaluation of Sensibility and Re-evaluation of Sensation in the Hand.* Baltimore: Williams and Wilkins, 1981.

Falk-Bergen A, Colangelo C. *Positioning the Client with Central Nervous System Deficits.* 2nd Edition. Valhalla Rehabilitation Publications, PO Box 195, Valhalla, NY 10595.

Holmes, D. The role of the occupational therapist in the work evaluation. *Am J Occupational Ther,* 39:5, 1985.

Healthcare Catalog. Fred Sammons, Inc. Box 32, Brookfield, IL 60513-0032.

Institute of Rehabilitation Medicine, New York University Medical Center and Campbell Soup Co. Mealtime Manual for People with Disabilities and the Aging. Box 56, Camden NJ 08101.

Mathiowetz V, Kashman N, Volland G, Weber K, Dowe M, Rogers S. Grip and pinch strength: normative data for adults. *Arch Phys Med Rehab* 66:69–74, 1985.

Mathiowetz V, Weimer DM, Federman SM. Grip and pinch strength: norms for 6–19 year olds. *Am J Occupational Ther* 40:705–711.

McCray P. *The Job Accommodation Handbook.* Verndale, MN: RPM Press, 1987.

North East Medical Inc. Catalogue, 187 Stauffer Blvd, San Jose, CA 95125-1042.

Trace Resource Book 1989–90 Edition. Assistive Technologies for Communication, Control and Computer Access. Trace Research and Development Center. Waisman Center, University of Wisconsin, Madison.

Trombly C, Scott A. *Occupational Therapy for Physical Dysfunction.* Baltimore: Williams and Wilkins, 1989.

Willard and Spackman's Occupational Therapy. 7th Edition. Philadelphia: JB Lippincott, 1988.

Wilson B, Moffat N. *Clinical Management of Memory Problems.* Aspen Publications, Rockville, MD.

Communication

Johns DR, Haynes S, Holland AL, LaPointe LL, Rosenbek JC, Wertz RT, Ylvisaker MS. *Clinical Management of Neurogenic Communcative Disorders.* San Diego: Little, Brown.

Dysphagia

Hargrove R. Feeding the severely dysphagic patient. *Am Assoc Neurosurg Nurses.* 12(2):102–107, 1980.

Hynak-Hankinson MR, Again M, Gardner C, Jones PL. Dysphagia evaluation and treatment: the team approach, part 1. *Nutritional Support Services* 4(5):33–41, 1984.

Logemann J. *Evaluation and Treatment of Swallowing Disorders.* College-Hill Press, Inc, San Diego, CA.

INDEX

P

Pain, in MS patients, 65–66
Paraspinal muscle treatment, 29
Pedestal base, 33
Pelvic tilt, 37
Pemoline, 75
Pharyngeal peristalsis, reduced, 118, 124, 127, 128, 129
Physical fitness, 56–57, 59; *see also* Exercise
Physical therapy, treatment structure, 19
Plantar flexion, 65
Plasticity, 39
Positioning, types, 27–29, 34
Positioning slant board, 20, 25
Preparatory posture, evaluation, 33
Pressure evaluation, for wheelchair cushions, 55
Purdue Pegboard, 73

Q

Quad set, 44

R

Range of motion, 15, 30, 72, 106–107
Recreation, issues for MS patients, 63; *see also* Specific types
Rehabilitation
  maintenance, 13–14
  restorative, 12–13, 14
Relaxation training, 38, 87–88, 89
Rhythmical rocking, 29
Rocker clog shoes, 52
Romberg test, 34

S

Sacral torsion, 65
Self-care, defined, 12; *see also* Specific types

Sensory feedback, 38, 47
Sensory impairment, 40, 136
  adaptations for
    bathing, 94
    dressing, 96
    eating, 97
    meal preparation, 99–100
    worksite,104–105
  evaluation, 68–69, 107
Shoulder abduction-adduction, 45
Shoulder flexion-extension, 44
Skiing, 64–65
Slow stroking, 29
Soft tissue shortening, 36
Spasticity
  compensating strategies for, in physical therapy, 19–20
  described, 17
  effect on coordination, 33
  effect on weakness, 40
  evaluation, 18–20, 73
  management
    cold packs, 30
    functional electric stimulation (FES), 30
    medication, 31
    movement techniques, 29
    pressure techniques, 29–30
    slow stroking, 29
  therapeutic exercises for, 20–27
Speech
  defined, 111
  evaluation, 112
  therapy, 115–116
    articulation exaggeration, 113
    compensated communication, 112
    echoing, 114
    nonverbal communication, 115
    pausing, 113

Notes

Notes

Notes

Notes